PENGUIN BOOKS

THE CHELSEA MURDERS

Lionel Davidson was born in Yorkshire in 1922 and now lives in Israel with his wife and two children. His first novel, *The Night of Wenceslas* (1960), won both the Crime Writers' Association prize for the best thriller of the year and the Authors' Club award for the most promising first novel. It was followed in 1962 by *The Rose of Tibet* and in 1966 by *A Long Way to Shiloh*, which was a Book Society Choice in Britain and a Book-of-the-Month Club Choice in the U.S.A. Mr Davidson's other highly praised novels are *The Sun Chemist, Smith's Gazelle* and *Making Good Again*.

LIONEL DAVIDSON

THE CHELSEA MURDERS

PENGUIN BOOKS

Penguin Books Ltd, Harmondsworth, Middlesex, England
Penguin Books, 625 Madison Avenue, New York, New York 10022, U.S.A.
Penguin Books Australia Ltd, Ringwood, Victoria, Australia
Penguin Books Canada Ltd, 2801 John Street, Markham, Ontario, Canada L3R 1B4
Penguin Books (N.Z.) Ltd, 182–190 Wairau Road, Auckland 10, New Zealand

—

First published in Great Britain by Jonathan Cape 1978
First published in the United States of America under the title
Murder Games by Coward, McCann & Geoghegan, Inc., 1978
Published in Penguin Books 1979

—

—

Made and printed in Great Britain by
Richard Clay (The Chaucer Press), Ltd,
Bungay, Suffolk
Set in Linotype Granjon

FOR YOSKE

One

She had three lilies
  in her hand
And the stars in her hair
  were seven.

I

In her black slip and her fluffy mules, Grooters was ironing a skirt. She was lumping around on the room's creaking floorboards to do this, in a state of high excitement. She had a date. She could scarcely remember when she'd had one last.

When the wardrobe door popped open, she shoved it to with her elbow and carried on ironing. But when it did it again she uttered an oath in Dutch and went hunting on the floor for the bit of paper that normally kept it shut.

One night the thing had creaked open just as she was going off to sleep, scaring her out of her wits. It had only been Penny fiddling in her own wardrobe at the other side of the locked partition door; but since then she'd kept it jammed.

She was on the top floor of the Comyns Hall of Residence, one of a group of student hostels in the Albert Bridge Road. Half the places at the Comyns were specifically for Chelsea students, of whom Grooters was one. She was studying sculpture at Chelsea Art School.

She found the paper and jammed the door, and as she did so felt further movement, which was strange. Penny had been away for a week. She was supposed to be away for another week.

She called, 'Penny?'

No answer from Penny's side; and no wonder. The girl couldn't hear her. Someone had a record-player blasting below.

Grooters had a quick peep through her curtains to see if light was coming from Penny's window, and it was, so that was all right; she had come back early.

She made fast work of the skirt and held it against her for a moment together with the new blouse that went with it, and looked in the wardrobe mirror. Now she'd done it, she wasn't sure the combination worked. As she pondered, her image came forward. To her astonishment, the whole wardrobe did, about three inches.

The door behind it had opened by the same amount.

Grooters's first thought was that it was a joke, and her second that she had better get the hell out of it. But she didn't fancy going downstairs in her slip.

She said, 'Is that you, Penny?'

The wardrobe moved a bit more. With her heart beginning to lurch, Grooters leaned hard against it and pushed it back. It didn't go all the way back; something had been wedged in the gap.

'That is you, Penny, isn't it?' Grooters said. But she was so frightened, the words hardly came out.

She knew it wasn't Penny.

She knew now that she had to get the hell out of it.

The safety catch was on the door. They had all been warned to keep their safety catches on lately.

She could feel her teeth chattering. With her back against the wardrobe, she reached out and pulled across the table she had been ironing on, and leaned against that, and then dragged the armchair over.

She tiptoed to the door in her mules, watching the wardrobe, and silently unchained the safety catch. She wanted to see the wardrobe move before she opened the door – to know that the person was at that end of the room and not this. It did move slightly. Everything moved – wardrobe, table, chair. Grooters opened the door and, with her legs turned to jelly, looked out.

The corridor was empty; everybody at dinner in the refectory. Elton John boomed up from the record-player below. She slipped her mules off and kicked them back in the room. Better in bare feet. On bare feet she crept past Penny's door, and saw the figure right away.

The figure saw her, too.

The door was open, and it stood in the middle of the room, arms away from its body.

It was very tall, with a large head, a woman's head. It wore a plastic cape and rubber boots and rubber gloves.

Grooters took in all this in one petrified glance and tried to scream. But she had never screamed well, and what came out was only a small moan. She found she was dancing from one foot to the other, unable to decide whether to make the dash to the stairs or to dash back. She didn't think she would make it to the stairs, so she scuttled back, her frantic idea being to lock herself into her small bathroom until people came back from the refectory.

She made it to her room and slammed the door, and then, as if in slow motion, every mini-second of the horror extending itself, realized that the figure had expected this. It had returned swiftly to the wardrobe, and with one lunge pushed it right in. With a rumble and a creak the wardrobe tottered, the table and chair both slid, and the thing was in the room with her.

The figure was so grotesque, Grooters felt her legs almost doubling underneath her, and she wet herself.

Despite the carnival character of the mask – curls piled high, open cupid's mouth radiantly smiling – the occupation suggested by the cape and the boots and gloves was rather that of a slaughterer, or a surgeon, perhaps even a mortuary attendant.

Grooters was a healthy young girl, and her training had strengthened her arms, but she had read of this apparition, and terror weakened her. She didn't make it to the bathroom, though she struggled quite hard, and she couldn't make it back to the door.

The figure twisted her round there, and got behind her, one arm crooking up round her throat. She heard the other one rustling in the plastic of the cape and presently felt, and choked on, the pad thrust over her mouth and nose.

She clawed to pull it away, but the arm that had been around her neck came up suddenly in a strong lock, reinforcing the one already in position. Grooters pummelled with her elbows and kicked with her bare feet, but she didn't do much damage and the pad wasn't even fractionally shifted.

She knew she mustn't breathe through the pad. The first sweetish smell had warned her. But she couldn't hold her breath for ever and, weeping, she knew she'd had it. She saw the room light begin first to spin slightly in her tears, and then recede along a familiar tunnel, together with Elton John.

Just for a moment before it all went, she knew she was only in the dentist's chair, and that it would all be all right, really. Then everything did go.

Feeling her succumb, her attacker waited a moment, and then lowered her to the floor, keeping the pad in place. One gloved hand felt in the large patch pocket of the cape, removing a plastic bag. Two rubber bands fell out. One went round the girl's face to keep the pad in position. Then the bag went over her head, and the other band secured it under her chin.

Grooters was left in this position, where she died presently, while her assailant went through to Penny's room and closed the outer door there. Returning, the murderer looked down at the girl and turned her over on her face; and then went into the small bathroom and turned on the shower and the water in the hand-basin.

Grooters remained where she was for a while, and then her murderer took off the bag. The rubber bands and pad went back in it, and everything was returned to the patch pocket, from which a small cleaver was removed. With this cleaver, the murderer proceeded to cut off Grooters's head.

The cleaver, of bluish steel and French make, had a small serrated portion. This dealt readily with the tough bits at the rear of the neck, and the rest presented no problem. A small tug and a slice released the head, and the murderer took it and put it face-down in the hand-basin, and went and stood under the shower.

This was about mid-way through the Chelsea murders.

It contained the elements that later identified the murderer; although this was no consolation to Grooters who by then was lying quietly in a cemetery in Leyden.

2

THREE weeks before, Artie was into murder. He was into blood that had sprayed on the ceiling. To have sprayed like that it could only have flicked back off a weapon striking an already bleeding wound.

'Jesus Christ,' he said.

He wrote it all down, though. He felt like bringing up.

The piece of gas-piping was grossly distorted and heavily bloodstained, Westminster Coroner's Court heard today. The bloodstains in the room, of a similar group to those found in Lord Lucan's car . . .

'I wonder if you would be so good,' said the old scholar next to him, rather breathlessly, 'as to keep your comments to yourself? I'd be awfully obliged.'

'No problem,' Artie said. He hadn't caught the old man's breathless stuff but he said 'no problem' on principle and carried on writing. Time was tight.

He was in Chelsea Reference Library.

Bloodstains on the ground floor were entirely Group A (Lady Lucan) apart from a tuft of bloodstained hair in the bathroom. But those in the Ford Corsair borrowed by Lord Lucan and found abandoned at Newhaven matched the groups of both Lady Lucan and murdered nanny Sandra Rivett.

He was high as a kite (bombed out of his mind, in fact; up all night and on Speed ever since) but he had an idea some chuffing was coming at him so he looked up. He found the old man mouthing at him with speechless rage. He had a healthy old face, pink skin, topped by silvery hair, but all of it was working. Artie had heard faces worked but had never before seen such a thing. This one was going like hell.

'You babble. You do nothing but babble,' the old man said, choking. 'You've babbled since you came. You have to keep silence here. It's impossible to concentrate on any work.'

Artie looked over to see what work he was concentrating on. It was *The Times* of 1875, and a magnifying glass was helping bring up the packed columns. Under the glass a small headline said *Mr Disraeli Purchases Suez Canal Shares.*

'Well, you just read the stuff I've got to read, Jack,' Artie told him, shaking his huge head, 'and you'd be babbling, too.'

Artie's stuff was hotter than Disraeli's. He had a pile of *Evening Standards* from June 1975.

'Don't be impudent. Don't call me Jack,' the old man said. His face was jerking so much he couldn't say any more. He shoved his volume along the desk, and joined it, and then shoved everything one place further. He looked back over the two empty

13

places, shaking. There was no healthy pink in Artie's skin, nor any trace of silver in his hair. All of him was black. His hair was an enormous globe of black. 'Damned insolence,' the old man said furiously at it.

'Just a saying,' Artie said.

He looked blindly out of the window. He knew he ought to have stayed in bed today. But there was too much to do, and he had promised Steve.

Now his eyes hurt and he felt himself trembling all over. He knew it was the Speed; he'd been gobbling the amphetamines for hours. The tablets kept the brain working but seemed to disconnect some other circuits. He could feel his brain up there, lodged like a pea in a pod.

Also the blood disgusted him today. It fascinated him, but mainly it was disgusting. How could it be green?

He wondered if they should make it red. But he knew they couldn't. Red was a piece of horseshit whatever you did. Red meant Hitchcock, with some girl going bananas every time she thought of blood. Or it meant psychedelic crap in various orders. It couldn't be red.

Anyway, they'd matched the green, a fabulous old green, very strange, very chemical. They were using it to show it was night-time. They had stolen a few frames from the Mary Pickford clip at the school. They planned to match the style of the 1920s captions, too, swelling and contracting like toads on the old acetate, bits crumbling off, blowing up bright then dim.

They'd agreed to use only one tint with the black and white; Steve, Frank, all of them had agreed. Frank was in charge of the art direction and he said the main thing was to stay away from the half-assed psychedelic areas. Artie certainly agreed with this, but he thought it was time now for Frank to offer some juice on the green blood question. Where the hell was Frank, anyway? He hadn't seen him all yesterday. He hadn't been on the location last night. Shouldn't he be here today?

He leafed through the rest of the needed stuff and tidied up.

He saw the chick on the desk smiling at him so he stopped there.

'You all done?' she said.

'Done done.'

'What's tomorrow – Jack the Ripper?'

'Right.' He threw her his most manic smile. Tomorrow was bed. All fugging day. 'Did Frank come in?' he said.

'I didn't see him.'

He looked beyond her to the Special Collections attic where Frank was mainly writing his book.

'He isn't up there, anyway,' she said.

He knew she didn't like Frank.

'Is he working some other place today?'

'What day is it – Wednesday?'

'I don't know what day it is. I don't know where the hell I am,' Artie said.

'Well, wow. You've been going it.'

She had a quaint cockney lilt and a dimple that showed as she smiled down at her hands. He saw he was supposed to notice the new thing she'd done with her hair. It gave her the look of a golden Pre-Raphaelite chick. Frank said they would all look that way after his book hit town.

'You could try across the road,' she said, nodding there.

'Maybe I will. Okay.'

He felt so disconnected going downstairs he thought he'd skip Frank. But out in the street he thought he wouldn't. A sudden shower had come smashing down. It was bouncing back off the road. The glass and concrete box of the art school, right opposite, looked as if newly formed there, steaming. The building depressed him always, but he ducked across to it.

He looked all over the lousy place but he couldn't find Frank, and scrambled out to Manresa Road again knowing he was late.

The rain had eased to a drizzle and he hunched through it to the corner. He had to grab a bus in the King's Road but when he got there he saw the whole street jammed with traffic, lines of buses stuck unmoving.

He began making it on foot, threading his way through the slanted umbrellas, hands over his head. He couldn't feel the rain but he knew it was there. He didn't want a headful of rain.

Now, in fresh air, moving, he felt disconnected from everything. Nothing was real, all Chelsea slanting with umbrellas, toytown. For minutes at a time he could hardly think why he was hurrying, or where. He passed a newspaper-seller on a corner and saw from a poster that someone had been murdered, but was well past before it meant anything.

He knew it couldn't be their murder. Their murder had been completed last night. He had taken everything back from it this morning, the costumes, the gear, everything. He'd returned the generator van, the lighting; dropped the cans of footage into the lab. All that was this morning; already another age.

He'd been awake forty hours. Another eight before he was through. He knew he needed more Speed, but he couldn't take it on an empty stomach. He'd eat first. He'd see Steve first.

The lights had come on everywhere. Going fast, not tiring, he passed rows of lighted boutiques, antique shops, restaurants, glistening in the rain. He turned in to Blue Stuff.

His spirits hit bottom in Blue Stuff. The place was packed with customers, come in out of the rain, damp and reeking. Mr Blue Stuff was there himself. The Chinaman had hardly any nose and no expression at all. He was telling a young fat girl how good she looked in a cowgirl jacket. All over the shop goons were fingering denim, shuffling through hangers, looking at themselves in it in mirrors. He saw Steve fitting an elderly one in a whole stiff suit of it. The scarecrow was holding his arms up at about forty-five degrees, a whimsical smile on his face, and Steve was tugging at him like a little pale gnome.

Steve looked frailer, more delicate than ever. Artie saw him leave the goon with his arms up and come over.

'You get it all back on time?' Steve said.

'Sure.'

'The genny, lights, everything?'

'No problem.' They hired on a daily basis. An hour after signing-in time and they'd hired for another day.

'How about the cans?'

'In. I made out the sheets. They know it's under-lit.'

'Great. You look shagged, Artie,' Steve said.

'Yeah. Anyway,' Artie said. He was tugging out his notes. 'Here's this. And we got problems with green blood. I was looking for Frank.'

'Leave Frank, Artie. He's low today.'

'I couldn't find him. Where the hell –'

'Leave him. It's that chick they pulled out of the river.'

'What chick?'

'Haven't you seen the news?'

'Jesus, I've had no time –'

'From The Gold Key. The barmaid. She's drowned. Leave him just for –'

'Hey, what you do?' Blue Stuff said. 'Customer standing.'

'Won't be a tick, Denny.' Blue Stuff's given name was Ogden, in honour of a Baptist minister in Hong Kong, but he was known as Denny, and on occasion Chairman, for he was also the chairman of his company, Wu Enterprises. He had a lot of enterprises, did Wu.

'No tick. Customer. What you want, Artie, you buy crose?'

'Just looking in, Denny.'

'Not a coffee shop. Flank rooking in, Arab rooking in. Crose shop here. Go somewhere else rook in.'

'Yeah, okay, only I've got to sleep tomorrow,' Artie told him, and realized he should be telling Steve. 'So don't call me,' he told Steve. 'I just brought this in. We can meet in the evening.'

'You're surely not going to work now.'

'I have to. I forgot to tell them I'd be up all night.'

'Rooking very fine. Extleme fashion,' Denny was saying as Artie left. He'd taken over the scarecrow himself, spreading his L's and R's as usual.

Artie was spreading his, too, as he went back out in the rain. Gleen blood. Why Flank in shop? Why Arab? He began to talk French to himself. He'd be speaking it for most of the evening. He could feel his brain tiring now. It was still going ceaselessly but it felt heavy. There was something it was trying to tell him, but it needed more Speed.

Before he got to work he passed another newspaper poster, however, and realized what it was. Strangled, the poster said. Drowned, Steve had said.

Could it be the same one? There were so many. Sleeping and waking, his life was full of murder lately.

'WHAT kind of beastly thing?' Mooney said. She was looking along her long legs and scruffy jeans to her sneakers, equally scruffy, on the arm of the next chair. (This was hours earlier and a couple of miles away.) There was no one else in the room and it was raining outside and she didn't feel very good, anyway. He'd asked her twice if he couldn't speak to the editor himself. She'd told him he couldn't. It was Wednesday, and the editor was off in Dorking putting the sodding thing to press.

She looked idly over the last proof pages, willing him to say 'contraceptive'. Not a bad little story if he'd gone and found one there in the vestry.

She saw she had quite a nice by-line on the front page. CHELSEA PENSIONER SAVES GIRL FROM GANG. *Gazette Reporter: Mary Mooney*. The phone on the next desk was giving her a headache, so she lifted it off. 'Vicar, could you hang on a tick,' she said, and answered it. 'News room.'

'Mary Mooney there?'

'Speaking . . . Chris?' she said. The *Evening Globe*.

'Mary – could you get down to The Gold Key, pub near World's End?'

'What's doing?'

'I don't know. Could be big. Germaine – check that spelling – Roberts. Barmaid. We've got it as Diane Germaine Roberts. She was picked up out of the river. A buzz from Scotland Yard. She was a part-timer there.'

'What, drowned?'

'Yeah, she was drowned. Packer was just on the blower. He's over there. Apparently she was living on the premises.'

'Gold Key. Germaine Roberts. Packer's where?' she said.

'At the Yard. He's staying there. The Gold Key is on the corner of –'

'I know The Gold Key. What – taxi?' Mooney said.

'Just get there fast as you can.'

'Okay, fine, I'll call,' Mooney said. She got her feet down off the chair. The *third*? Was it possible? 'Hello, sorry, Vicar,' she said. 'Urgent call there. Can I ring you back later?'

'Well, I wonder if the editor could –'

'Of course,' Mooney said. 'I'll see he gets the message. I'll make a special point of it.'

She shot off down the stairs and got her bike. It was in the narrow passage at the foot of the stairs next to the advertising department. There was hardly room to squeeze it in and they always kicked up a row. She'd told them, the best thing was to widen the passage. She wasn't leaving it outside. She got her plastic off the hanger and wound it round her. She hated the shitty place. A regular little artisan's cottage.

They'd been kicked out of the King's Road, together with the *Chelsea News*, after seventy years. The leases had fallen in. Boutiques had taken over at twelve times the rent. The same thing was happening all over Chelsea. Now they were chronicling events (to give the activity a name) from the middle of Fulham. All the management had done was tart up the ground floor with plate glass and carpets and a rubber plant and put a sign over the top, CHELSEA GAZETTE. It looked like a poofish dry-cleaner's or a travel agency. The editorial, above, remained in its pristine squalor. Never mind.

She trundled her vehicle out to the street, and slammed the side door behind her. She'd save on a taxi (60p there and 60p back, with any understanding at the *Globe* end), and it would be quicker by bike, anyway.

Mooney was six feet tall and thirty years old, a divorcee. She had a heavy long Spanish face which attracted the wrong kind of person. She knew about this as about a lot of things. Her journalistic career had been interrupted by marriage and motherhood (and divorce and bereavement, respectively), and she had since learned to cope with a number of problems, including the contraction of the Fleet Street Press which made it difficult for her to get a job there. She had returned to her first job on the *Chelsea Gazette*, at minimum rates, turning a penny here and there with extras as a stringer for the London Press, a lot of which involved getting rain in your face.

She turned in before World's End at Stanley Street, with The Gold Key on the corner, and right away saw the fuzz flexing outside.

'Morning,' she said politely, wheeling her cycle and standing it outside the Gents'. 'I wonder if I could ask you to keep an eye on that.'

The constable didn't say anything, but when he saw her going to the side door and pressing the bell, he came up to her.

'What did you want?' he said.

'Mr Logan,' she said. She'd suddenly remembered the name from the little gilt sign above the door, *Gerald Logan, Licensed to sell Beers, Spirits, Wines & Tobaccos*.

'Oh, yes?' the constable said.

In one joyous burst she realized that nobody had got here yet. 'Gerry,' she said.

'Was it anything special?' the constable said.

The door opened and a skinny little woman in an overall was standing there.

'Hello, dear,' Mooney said, nodding most warmly. She'd never cast eyes on her before. 'Tell him I'm here. It's Mrs Mooney.'

The woman and the constable were both looking at her anxiously.

'I came the moment I could,' Mooney apologized.

After looking anxiously at her, the fuzz and the help were now looking at each other. 'How *is* he?' Mooney said. An advantage of her heavy eyes and long Spanish chops was that, despite her gangling figure, she could transform at will into Our Lady of Sorrows. 'In a dreadful state, I'm sure.'

'Well, he is,' the help said. She was scratching at a little wart on her lip. 'Just a minute, I'll see.' She looked nervously at the constable and went.

'What, er, actually was it?' the fuzz said.

'It's at times like these,' Mooney said, dropping him a look of bottomless compassion, 'that we're really needed.' While dropping him it she uneasily recalled having seen him knocking about the area. He didn't seem to have recalled her yet, which was something.

'I'm not supposed to let anyone in, you see,' he said.

'Not even *us*?' Mooney said, incredulously.

Logan was suddenly standing there. She remembered him when she saw him, big beery belly, potato face. 'Oh, Gerry!'

'Yeah. Jesus,' he said. 'Who is it?'

'What can I say to you?' Mooney said, solemnly pushing him inside. 'The shock of it!'

'Yeah,' Logan said again. He was watching with bemusement as she closed the door in the constable's face. 'I don't know what the hell is happening,' he said.

'Of course you don't, poor man,' Mooney told him. 'You can carry on now,' she said to the help.

Mooney didn't know how all this commanding stuff was coming out of her. It rose unbidden at moments of creation, such as the dawn of a truly shit-hot story. There was one here. She had absolutely no doubt about it. Fuzz at the door – for a common drowning? Not likely. Something was going on. Better still, it was just one piece of fuzz, unconfident of instructions, not totally in possession of his marbles. Surely a rapid drafting from an undermanned local station? He was holding the fort till the C.I.D. men arrived. They hadn't arrived yet. She was in at the dawn.

'Let's go to her room,' she said, realizing the mileage that had to be crammed into a few minutes. She was on tenterhooks for the sound of a siren.

'Her room?' Logan said.

'Germaine.'

'Germaine's room?'

'Poor man, you're all done in,' Mooney said, suppressing an urge to do him in. His hair was dishevelled, wits all away. This was the way they had to be kept. 'You lead the way,' she said. 'I'll need to contact her dear parents.'

'Germaine's parents? What parents?' Logan said.

'The rest of her poor family,' she amended. No parents. Or the girl was a liar. What was a part-timer doing *living* on the premises, anyway? The place smelt terrible, unaired, and only half an hour to opening time. Where was the landlady? Something was amiss here, the story improving by the moment. They were standing in a dark beery little porch, one passage leading to the cavernous bar, another to inner regions. She turned there. 'I think I remember it,' she said.

'No, let me,' Logan said. 'What was that name – Mooney?'

'Mooney. *Mary*,' she gently reproved.

'Sorry, Mary. This is a hell of a thing. Are you a relation, then?'

'Not a *relation*,' Mooney said, again reprovingly. 'I'll have to tell her relations . . . So full of life. What happened?'

'I don't know what happened.' Logan's enormous backside, flapping shiny cloth, sagged ahead of her up the steep stairs. 'She said she didn't feel well. She came up here about nine o'clock. We had a full house.'

'You gave her a knock.'

'I gave her a knock,' Logan agreed. 'I don't know when, maybe half-past, and she said she'd come down, but she never.'

No landlady, then; and he hadn't sent anyone else up to give her a knock. Logan was in the way of giving her knocks. All good.

'And later she wasn't there?' Mooney said.

'That's right,' Logan said, and looked round at her with his mouth open. 'Were you here, then?' he said.

Mooney sorrowfully shook her head, and solicitously prodded his rear upwards. She had an acute mental image of police cars coming down the King's Road at this very minute; also of assemblies of taxis en route from Fleet Street, occupants' eyes fixed on the meters.

It wasn't on the first landing. Germaine's room was an attic. A frowsty one, too; the deceased, on the immediate evidence, a first-class slut. There was a heavy female smell in the curtained room. The bed had been slept in and hastily made up again, covers thrown over. A few shoes were kicked under a small padded chair, on which was a tangle of tights and of grotty, by no means spotless, knickers; Germaine not a big, or regular, washer.

A combful of blondish hair was on a dressing table whose glass top was finely dusted with powder. Under the glass was a selection of photos; one, squarish and larger than the others, of a pony-tailed blonde looking candidly up from some undisclosed activity on a floor. Enormous boobs drooped from a bikini top. A quarter page, Mooney hungrily thought, if ever she'd seen one. If it happened to be old Germaine, of course ... She sought frantically for ways to pose her inquiry.

'Is this recent?' she said reverently.

'I don't know when she had it done,' Logan said moodily.

'Ah, they will love it,' Mooney said; she raised the glass and whipped the thing out. On the back, to her still dawning astonishment at the nature of what was blossoming here, a rubber stamp said *Property of the I.L.E.A.* She had it in her shoulder bag in a flash. 'It reminds me so of her last holiday,' she said, shaking her head. 'Things go so fast, when was it now?'

She had thought, with the impregnated air of the room, that Logan was about to sneeze, but realized, with no loss of faculties, that he was crying. 'Perhaps her passport will tell us,' she said.

*

She called the *Globe* from a call-box two hundred yards away, having thanked the fuzz for looking after her bike. She heard the sirens going as she got through.

'Chris, you're right, it's a big one. Anything fresh from Packer, first?'

'Yeah. She was strangled. The river police picked her out downstream of Albert Bridge but she must have gone in between Wandsworth and Battersea, maybe Lots Road. Don't mess about, love, what have you got?'

'What I've got, first of all, is a fantastic picture. Exclusive.'

'Portrait?'

'*Portrait?* Tits down to here. Bikini.'

'Yeah?'

'It looks professional.' She was gazing at it. 'It says I.L.E.A. on the back. That's something, eh?'

'I.L.E.A.?'

'Inner London Education Authority.'

'What does that mean?'

23

'Well, damn it, what can it mean? An art school. She was modelling. We haven't just got a barmaid here. We've got an artist's model. Murdered. In Chelsea.'

'Christ. Anybody else got it?'

'Nobody. I was there before the C.I.D. I can hear them now. There are sirens going. Listen, I'll bring it in. I'd better give you a bit of stuff first.'

'Okay, hang on. I'll put you on to Typists.' The phone jiggled. 'Transfer this call to copy-takers. Urgent.'

'Copy,' Typists said.

'Mooney, Chelsea,' Mooney said.

'Yeah, Mary.'

'Chelsea Art Model Murder.'

'Chelsea Art Model Murder,' Typists said, clicking away.

'Distraught fifty-four-year-old Gerald Logan, landlord of The Gold Key,' Mooney dictated. She spelled it out. She spelled out the girl's name, too, and her age, and all the other passport details. She spelled out about fifty-four-year-old Gerald's wife, now dying in the Brompton Hospital, and how he had given the twenty-five-year-old Manchester hopeful bed and board while she pursued her promising career.

Fifty-four-year-old Gerald and twenty-five-year-old Germaine had both liked a breath of river air before packing it in for the night. Not finding her, he had gone to see if she was taking one by herself. He wondered if she had strolled over to the opposite bank where he had seen some television or film shooting going on at one of the abandoned wharves, but he hadn't gone to see.

'You want that last par in?' Typists said. There had been some trouble unscrambling it.

'Why not? I've got a photo-caption, too,' Mooney said. 'Do you want it?'

'Who's got the photo?'

'I have. I'm bringing it in.'

'No, love. Art department, when you get here.'

'Mooney, Chelsea, right?'

'Got it.'

4

THE men making the siren noise spent some minutes clearing up the mystery of Mrs Mooney. There were mysteries in abundance already but to Detective Chief Inspector Summers one of the biggest was how a young prick like this constable on the door had ever got into the force.

'What's your name, son?' he said.

'Nutter,' the constable said, reddening.

'Yes.' The chief inspector let it hang in the air. *Well, I don't want to be hard on you, lad*, were the words that sprang to mind but he left them unuttered. With a name like that a lifetime of problems lay ahead, anyway. 'And you thought she was what?' he said.

'Well, a nun, something like that.'

'In jeans?' (*On a bike? Mrs?*)

'*Something* like that. A missionary, or a welfare worker, something religious. They expected her here. I thought they did, sir. She told *them* that,' he said aggrievedly.

This seemed to be the case. The help said she'd thought the landlord had phoned her. The landlord said he'd thought someone had sent her. They were all standing in the beery little porch looking at each other. The landlord didn't seem to know his arse from his elbow; for which, the chief inspector thought, there might be good reasons. He had a recent piece of information which he wished to pursue, so he said, 'Let's get on, then. You lead the way, landlord. Take over here, Mason,' he added with a significant look at Nutter.

Detective Constable Mason took poor Nutter outside.

'Never mind him,' he said. 'We all make mistakes.'

'Yes, don't we?' Nutter said, his colour still high. He didn't like references to his name. 'And some go on making them,' he added.

Mason understood the allusion; common lately. But all he said was, 'That's what makes him irritable.'

'Well, people in glass houses,' madly persisted Nutter.

Yeah, okay, Nutter. You toddle off then, Nutter. You'll be all right, Nutter, old son, was what Mason passionately wanted to urge the fool. But again he held off, only nodding as Nutter strode proudly away. With a name like that, the plain-clothes man thought, strategy was needed, and Nutter didn't seem to have any.

Mason had plenty himself. He was a very controlled young man, a promising detective. He had an idea something promising was doing here.

Logan's sagging behind was meanwhile once more making the dolorous ascent to Germaine's bower; and within about five minutes he was crying again. There was no opening time at The Gold Key that morning, though a growing band of customers – augmented by thirty ladies and gentlemen of the Press – impatiently awaited it.

*

The girl had been murdered; the third murder in a fortnight, and the third within a mile.

The man stuck with this bad news sat sourly in his room, one of a suite he'd taken over at Chelsea police station as his Murder HQ, and realized he was in the deep end again.

(He didn't yet know how deep. The girl without the head still had it that morning; she had some time to go with it.)

His name was Warton and he was a detective chief superintendent, a powerful roly-poly figure who seemed below medium height because of his enormous barrel chest and hunched shoulders. He had very little neck and a round baldish head which protruded outwards into an immensely long snout. It gave him the appearance of a wart-hog.

By nature and training Warton was an unpleasant man; suspicious, close-grained, unfriendly. He was very senior in his job, which for a long time now had been striking him as a ridiculous one; it seemed high time he was out of it and into something more solid and administrative with set hours and respectable anonymity. There was something raffish and unsavoury in this skittering about, setting up headquarters and solving mysteries.

However, he was better than competent at it, which was why he was here.

When the first murder had occurred the newly appointed Crime Commissioner (C.C.) at the Yard had immediately sent for one of his commanders and said, 'Get someone reliable on this right away, someone like Ted Warton. We can't have a nonsense here.'

There'd been too many nonsenses. There had been the nonsense involving Lord Lucan, and Lady Lucan. There had been the nonsense with Slipper of the Yard, returned from Brazil without his rightful captive, Biggs the train-robber. There had been the Cambridge rapist who had terrorized the university town for months until on his belated, almost accidental, capture he had been found to have a record from here to next week apart from having left prodigal evidence, including signed messages, in his trail.

None of this was good for the police.

'What's Ted got on his plate?' the C.C. had inquired.

Warton had nothing. He had been cunningly clearing things off his plate in anticipation of translation to other sees. This was how he had bought the assignment.

Two weeks before, an American called Alvin C. Schuster had been found wrapped round a lamp-post near his house in Bywater Street. There were two stab wounds in his chest and he had been dead for three hours.

A neighbour exercising her dog had first noticed him at a few minutes to midnight. Other neighbours had been stepping in and out of their houses all evening without having noticed him, which had brought Warton out in his first evil distemper.

Obviously, someone had put Schuster round that lamp-post – and shortly before the neighbour found him. This wasn't an easy thing to do, unless Schuster had been dragged there from his house. This he had not been. The family dog never failed to bark when Schuster so much as approached the house. It hadn't barked.

But if he hadn't reached the lamp-post via his house, how had he got there? Bywater Street was a cul-de-sac lined bumper-to-bumper with the cars of the residents. It could only be entered from the King's Road; getting to the lamp-post, which was three-quarters of the way down it, would have caused considerable commotion even by sedan chair.

Warton's frazzled inquiries into any possible Intelligence angle – result negative – had brought him an early morning call, at home, from the C.C. He had been curtly told not to put funny buzzes about. The Americans leaked things, and people talked. The C.C. told him to remember the people he had in the district, and to treat the case as one of normal murder.

Warton knew the people he had in the district – troublemakers of all kinds, judges, bankers, politicians. Mrs Margaret Thatcher, the leader of the Conservative Party, had her well-publicized abode in Flood Street, just a few hundred yards from Schuster's lamp-post.

He also knew normal murder. Long grubby experience taught that ninety-nine per cent of it was domestic in origin.

However, it didn't seem to be the origin in Schuster's.

So far as the most thorough investigation could show, Alvin C. had been having no side orders of sex; no arguments, either, or drink or drugs, or any other kinds of trouble. He had been a cheery horn-rimmed oil executive, sensitive to the anxieties of labour in industry, mindful of the role of management. He owed nobody any money. Nobody owed him any. He hadn't sacked anybody much.

Warton thought the most likely thing was that someone had got the wrong bloke.

Unfortunately, this was worse than getting the right one. Your average bloke, reading his paper, could well understand how even the most violent and baffling of murders had a rational cause. A natural justice or reason would be found lurking beneath the surface of the thing. Wrong blokes were a different kettle of fish entirely. Anybody could turn out to be one of those. It led to anxiety and indignation, and often letters to legislators (many living in Chelsea).

He had proceeded from the phone call to his Chelsea HQ (unpromisingly sited in Lucan Place) immediately into the next golden spot of the day. His deputy, Summers, had greeted him with the news that they had got another. Two streets away from Schuster, Jubilee Place, a daily had shown up with a bright good morning to find her employer starkers in the hall. Her employer had been Miss Jane Manningham-Worsley, aged 82. She had been throttled and raped.

Warton went to the third floor flat and had a look at her.

Everything was in ship-shape order (saving Miss Manningham-Worsley) except that the daily said the safety catch wasn't on. She had never known it not to be on unless the old lady had admitted a friend. This meant that the old lady had had an aberration, or that she had known and admitted the friend who had raped and throttled her, or that the bastard had come in some other way.

Nothing of value was missing; not the old lady's money, not any of her jewellery. The only thing the daily couldn't find was a jar of pickles she had brought the day before.

Warton felt his subordinates looking at him so he lit a cigarette and went down to the car and hunched there, looking more of a wart-hog than ever.

Yes. All as normal. All they wanted in this one was a chap with a zest for pickles and for ladies of 82.

No sense anywhere. Not a glimmer of it.

He had depressively told his wife so, as he'd wound the clock last night at Sanderstead.

But long before the clock rang, his bedside phone did.

Four in the morning.

Summers's voice was hushed at the other end.

'Thought you'd want to know, sir. River police have a floater in our patch.'

'Right.'

He had lumbered up at once and out to the car in the dark.

He'd stood hunched at the autopsy, simply nodding as the pathologist pointed silently to the bruised Adam's apple.

'Anything doing?' he asked.

The pathologist manipulated Germaine a bit.

'Oh, I think so,' he said.

'Okay. Open her.'

The first moment of true satisfaction in a couple of weeks had come when the midget foetal mess was cupped invitingly for his attention in the pathologist's glove.

'How old's that?'

'Ten weeks? I could tell you better tomorrow.'

'Fine.'

So it was. Sense at last! Two people had been involved in the making of that gloveful. Find the other, he'd found his lead.

'He didn't know *what*?' he therefore demanded menacingly now of Summers. Summers had just returned from The Gold Key.

'That she was pregnant, sir. I'd go bail on it.'

'But having it off with her?'

'Oh, not a doubt of that.' Unlike his boss, the chief inspector was a tall and gaunt individual, a pipe-smoking bloodhound. 'All I can say, is that he seemed surprised to me. Shocked. Taken aback,' he amended.

'Chaps having it off get taken aback when young women are put in the club?'

'Days of the pill, sir.'

'Which she was on, was she?'

'Evidently not.'

'*Evidently* not. What the hell are you on about, Summers?'

'Well, sir.' Summers tamped his pipe. 'The thing with this girl – I've got a few lines out – she was a bit of an all-rounder. Both sexes, general fun and games.'

'I can tell you one game, Summers,' Warton said, inner eye constant on the only bit of sense these past two weeks, 'and one sex that put her in the club. Know which one?'

'My meaning there,' Summers said mildly, 'was that given her way of life, it wouldn't have caused much alarm. I'd guess she'd had a spot of trouble before, sir, wouldn't you?'

Warton declined to speculate on other trouble.

He sat hunched and brooding over his own.

'This landlord. Weeper,' he said. 'Just as untroubled, is he?'

'He's over the top,' Summers said briefly. 'Petrified his wife will find out – result of this case. Dying in hospital. You'll see it there, sir.'

Warton grunted, examining the papers placed on his desk.

'What's this film crew over the river?' he said.

'Semi-amateur crew. We'll have more later.'

'Who's Mrs Mooney?'

'Yes.' Summers began scraping his pipe. 'Slight cock-up there. Uniformed man on the door let her in before we got there. Some confusion about what she wanted.'

'Bike. Jeans,' Warton read out. 'That's a local reporter,' he said, looking sharply up.

Summers scraped away. 'What I thought,' he said.

So he had, after Detective Mason had diffidently suggested it.

'She'll be a stringer. For one of the nationals.' Warning bells had begun to clamour in Warton's brain. 'Before you got there . . .? What did she get, then?'

'Well, the landlord was a bity hazy as to exactly –'

'What was there to get? What have we got? What was she doing, this part-timer, when not at the bar or having her fun?'

'A bit of modelling, nothing very –'

'What – masseuse?'

'No. Just the odd session posing for –'

'A model? An *artist's* model? A real Chelsea artist's model?'

A certain baying note in his voice, an experienced old note, brought the inspector's startled face up from his pipe.

'You could call it that,' he admitted with quiet alarm.

'*Could* call it? They bloody will, bet your bottom dollar. Did she get a photo? Were there any photos?'

'Well, a few snapshots, but I don't think –'

There was a polite knock on the door. 'Latest editions, sir.'

With a wordless snarl Warton had them on his desk.

The *Evening News* and the *Standard* had sizeable headlines: CHELSEA BARMAID MURDERED, and a photo of The Gold Key.

The *Globe* had a much more sizeable headline: CHELSEA ART MODEL MURDERED, also a photo of The Gold Key: also another one, a huge one, flagged *Exclusive*, of Germaine looking candidly up from a floor.

Just a few short hours before, the superintendent had seen her looking up from a slab. He read through the big type of the intro, and the columns underneath, and on the back. Playing it up big.

Twenty-five-year-old Germaine ... feeling unwell ... in the nude for life classes at Chelsea Art School ... registered as a model with the Inner London Education Authority ...

He knew from a slight stiffening behind him exactly when Summers connected with that. A bit of posing, just the odd session, eh? Bloody newspapers had it, and the police didn't. Should have had it: model, looking for work, Chelsea. Warton stored this in his festering brain bank and read on.

They actually had a little picture of him, on page 2, looking like a tit in a trance as he had emerged from Miss Jane Manningham-Worsley's to have a drag in the car while pondering the pickles in the earlier nightmare. *Det. Ch. Supt. Edward Warton, in charge of the Chelsea Inquiries*, read the caption, and an accompanying small box encapsulated the nature of the inquiries to date.

Yes. All they weren't using were phrases like 'tight-lipped police officials were not indicating today whether ...'

There were certain phrases that catastrophes to others had taught him to watch out for. They weren't using this one yet. They hadn't got on to the pregnancy, either. They were sniffing at it. 'Feeling unwell.' Sniffing at it.

There was a lot he had to say to Summers, and the moment he looked at Summers he knew that Summers was expecting it, but he didn't say it yet. That was not his way.

'They haven't got the pregnancy yet, Summers,' was all he said.

'No, sir.'

'I don't want them to.' Summoning huge reserves he said, 'You could be right, Summers. He might not have anything to do with it. But somebody had. He's not answering calls, is he?'

'No, we've got someone there, sir.'

Warton sat brooding. It was hours since he'd stumbled out in the dark. He had a longing for a nice stressless office; desk, central carpet, smell of floor polish. Problems to do with manning, budgets, the odd conference. Might bring in a few flowers from the garden at Sanderstead. Decent neighbours there, insurance officials, bank officials. See them getting up in the middle of the night to examine the inside of a whore.

His mouth was well furred, but he lit a cigarette and broodingly examined the box on page 2 again. It had the quality of a tombstone. He scented something about it. It might not have occurred to them yet; they worked fast and were mainly in the dark, too.

'Summers, you and I know these murders have nothing in common, don't we?'

'Obvious, sir.' Summers relaxed slightly.

'Ng.' Warton drew on his cigarette. 'One of these bright bastards, give him a day or two, will start asking if we haven't got a maniac here.'

5

'THINK we've got a maniac here, Chris?'

'Maniac, h'm.'

'What do you think?'

'Maniac. Strong.'

'Not bad, though, is it?'

'Oh, not *bad*. No. Maniac.'

'Chelsea maniac,' the editor said.

'Chelsea maniac.'

They sampled it a bit, looking at each other.

'I'm wondering if we've quite reached that point,' Chris said.

'Well, have they reached some other?'

'Oh, no. Running about. Still, the elements are a bit mixed, aren't they? American oil man. Eighty-two-year-old spinster. Barmaid.'

'Model,' the editor said.

'Model,' Chris allowed.

'Was she in the pudding club, by the way?'

'Probably. They aren't saying.'

'What's the landlord say?'

'He isn't saying. You can't get at him.'

'What about friends?'

'We're trying friends. Mooney is.'

'Yes. Good work from her. Bonus, I think.'

'Thanks. She'll be glad. What she's really after,' Chris said, 'is a job.'

'I know. Tricky, that. Hiring problems and so forth.'

'Oh, sure . . . I mean, I get the *story*. It's strong, though.'

'I like it,' the editor said, simply.

'I like it, too.'

'It's a very good word. As a word.'

'Oh, good word.'

'With follow-through . . . Bed-sitters, student hostels, old-age homes.'

'Judo, karate, manly arts.'

'Double locks, peep-holes . . . I basically wanted *you* to be convinced there was stuff, Chris.'

'Well, I am, Jack,' Chris said. 'Womanly arts, too, come to that,' he added. 'Special evening classes. They get them going for the balls, don't they?'

'And that spray. What's that spray stuff?'

'Mace.'

'That. Run on the stocks. Suppliers besieged . . . You know, it's a little beauty when you think of it. Gun licences, dogs. Dogs good. What was that word a moment ago? Besieged. Chelsea besieged.'

'Chelsea Under Siege.'

'I'll think of it. Good night shot. Policeman watching. Atmospheric. Damn it, it's better than Cambridge! Well, it's Chelsea, isn't it? Double locks, peep-holes. And the Thatcher angle – never let us forget. Copper watching Thatcher. Anyone can get raped, can't they? Jesus,' he said, wistfully.

'Yeah. I mean, it's good, anyway,' Chris said. 'We're working on this film crew. You know, filming while it actually happened. They seem to have a spade in charge.'

'Really?'

'Yeah, real one, all black. Johnston. Artie Johnston,' he said, looking at a note. 'Nominal producer. Some arty-farty thing. Using various gilded Chelsea layabouts. Opens up certain vistas.'

'Yes. Who else have they got?'

'Director a young kook, Steve – is it? – yes, Giffard, brilliant career at film school, great things expected. The whole thing is kooky. It's a group. What I was thinking there – the Polanski case, gifted director, wife murdered, the Manson shower. You know. Also, the art director's a lecturer at Chelsea Art School – could easily have known this girl.'

'Who is he?'

'Another weirdo. Frank – *Doctor* Frank Colbert-Greer. Art historian. Queer as a coot. He's writing a book on something.'

'Where's this from – Mooney?'

'Yeah. What I was thinking – they're all young. Gifted. *Evil*, is what I was sort of straining away at. A kind of nest, or *coven*. Know what I mean?'

'Yes. I wouldn't go overboard, though. I mean, I get the angles – evil, covens, gifted young. On the other hand, it isn't a maniac, is it?' asked the editor seriously. 'Get one of those on his rounds and you can't print enough copies. Women going in fear. What's the bastard up to? They seek him here, they seek him there. Panic stalks the streets. Closely followed by us.'

'Well, I see that, but –'

'Not for a moment that I'm pissing on covens. It's simply a question of proportion. There ought to be some way of speeding this up. They aren't getting tight-lipped yet, are they?'

'Not yet. Not really. Only on whether she was in the club or not. Understandable.'

'Yes. Don't let's be too understanding ... Greer. I've heard of him.'

'The father. Portraitist. Painted all the Bloomsbury group. Dr Frank's the fruit of his late fornications.'

'Got him, have we?'

'We will. He's out of sight at the moment.'

'What do you mean, out of sight?'

'Not at home. Gone away.'

'Police looking for him?'

'We are.'

'What's this, Chris?'

'Little hunch of Mooney's. There might be nothing in it. She gets things, that girl, though.'

6

MOONEY was just then getting the beer. She was doing it in The Chelsea Potter (known as The Potters), one of a dozen pubs in the stretch between Sloane Square and World's End. The attraction of The Potters was that Frank regularly used it. It didn't look as if he'd be doing so tonight, however. All she'd got was Artie and Steve.

'Well, then,' she said, making the best of this. 'And how's Frank and his book these days? Where is he, anyway?'

'Frank?' Steve said. 'Well, I think he's just about up to Rossetti – that it, Artie?'

'Rossetti?' Artie said, startled. 'Oh, *Rossetti*. Dante Gabriel. Big Gabe,' he added. 'Yeah, that's where he's at with it.'

'Well, good,' Mooney said.

Something was going on, for certain. No questions were being answered on Frank. She tried again.

'It's time I gave him another par on that, I promised him. There ought to be a way I could tie up the book with the film, give you all a turn.'

'Sweetheart, it's not a Pre-Raphaelite *film*,' Artie told her.

He was like a long black cat, golliwog smile in place under his beehive; she smiled back at him.

'How did the night-shooting go, incidentally?'

'Good. You should have come. I told you.'

'Does *Frank* take a practical interest in that?' she asked with immense seriousness.

'Well, of course he does. He has to,' Artie said. 'There's a hundred things, costume, period, style.'

'He was there, was he?'

She actually saw Steve's foot move there, just as Artie opened his mouth. Artie didn't falter. 'Well, that's always a scramble,' he said. 'I've got to keep my eyes on everything to be sure we don't miss things. I mean, we hire that stuff practically by the minute. Well, you know how we're working.'

Mooney knew how they were working. She'd done a couple of stories on the film, which she'd thought at first a joke. She knew now it was no joke. They were obsessed with it. Every penny they had or could borrow had gone into it. They'd taken their dim part-time jobs just to be able to carry on with it.

She listened as Artie carried on about it now: their hand-cranking flicker effects, the long mascara looks, bumbling Keystone cops – all the 1920-ish tricks they were using to make a piece of period slapstick out of some contemporary situations.

She'd heard it all before, though, so she watched Steve.

She saw that the little manikin, though relaxed, was watching her. It was his idea, most of the film, she knew. He'd dreamed it up at the film school. All three of them, Steve, Artie and Frank, had been at the school – and before that at Chelsea Art School. Frank was back at the art school now, though as a lecturer this time.

She sought for ways to get back to Frank; and tackled it her own way, as soon as Artie drew breath.

'How's Abo, then?' she said. 'Still coming up with the bread?'

The foot moved again, and this time Artie did falter.

'Why – I guess so,' he said.

'Of course he is,' said little Steve. 'That's a *bright* Arab.'

'What's he doing these days?'

'Shagging his ears off,' Artie said.

'Apart from that.'

What Abo was doing apart from that, as Mooney knew, was learning English, with Frank.

'I haven't seen too much of him,' Steve said.

'Has he got over that cousin of his?'

'Unfortunately.'

'Some party!'

'It was.' Steve sipped his beer. 'What that Arab needs is more cousins.'

'I thought he had two thousand already,' Artie said; adding curiously, 'And why the hell is every last one of them called Feisal?'

'They aren't,' Mooney said. 'Some are called Abo.'

'Well, that's right,' Artie confessed. 'And Mohammed. Abo is a Mohammed, too.'

'No, he isn't.' Mooney was the expert on this. She had written a little piece after Abo's commemorative party for his young countryman Feisal, who had been beheaded for assassinating his Uncle Feisal, king of Saudi Arabia. 'He's *ibn* Mohammed – Abdul Azbig *ibn* Mohammed. It means his father was Mohammed.'

'Every Arab's father was Mohammed,' Steve said. 'He was the father of the race.'

'No, he wasn't.' Mooney knew this, too. 'Abraham was. He was the father of all the Semites, Jews *and* Arabs.'

'Catholic guy, Abraham. Ibrahim,' Steve said prissily, speaking like Abo.

Just then Abo spoke for himself. 'Hello,' he said, with muted delight. He'd swung in, questing, from the King's Road, long leather jacket swinging. Mooney recollected the boom of a Ferrari some moments before.

'Hello, Abo, we were discussing your Catholic family,' she said.

'Catholic?'

'Have a beer,' Mooney said.

'Whisky. Whisky?' Abo said, producing his wallet.

'Go on, pervert us.'

Abo bought the whisky, sizing up the form in the pub. There wasn't much; Thursday evening. The labourers who favoured the place were paid on Friday. Abo, twenty years old, weirdly resembling in feature his late monarch Feisal, had catholic tastes.

'I've been meaning to call you, Abo,' Mooney said, in a friendly fashion. In her many calls today she'd already tried him a dozen times. 'How's it going?'

'Very good.'

'How are the English studies?'

'Good,' Abo said.

'How's Frank?'

'He is my good friend.'

'Teaching you much English?'

38

'Much. Oh!' Abo said, rolling his eyes to show how much.

'Did he work you hard today?'

'Not today. Frank not here today.'

'Where is he?'

'We fold our tents,' Steve said, 'and quietly steal away. Longfellow.'

'So soon?'

'Artie has a job,' Steve said, 'which I'm walking him to. But we'd be glad of a piece. Really. Let's get together soon.'

'Sure,' Mooney said, and hungrily watched them go.

Nothing out of Abo, as she'd instantly sensed. He didn't know anything. That was why they'd left her with him.

All Abo knew (though he bought her another whisky) was that this was one of the ugliest women he'd ever seen. Women should be blonde and about his own size, which was five foot five, and they should have faces either like dolls or like gazelles. This one had a face like a camel.

But he thought his own thoughts, and Mooney thought hers.

She thought about Artie.

He was weird.

They all were, but he was possibly the weirdest. There couldn't be too many young Liverpool blacks who'd translated and published their own versions of the poems of Rimbaud. She knew about his sea-going days, of his three years in Paris and two in Los Angeles; his art school scholarship. Now he was producer of the film, and it was in this capacity, as she knew, that he was reading away in the reference library, covering all the cases in which the police had made particular fools of themselves – both to duplicate the hairier bits of action and to steer them clear of libel.

Knowing all this, she still felt she didn't know much.

She knew far more about Frank, if only because feckless Frank told you everything – even his most 'intimate' items. He'd had lectureships at several art schools until he'd decided suddenly to do his book on the Pre-Raphaelites, and had then dropped the other schools, retaining only Chelsea.

To make ends meet and pay his whack with the film, he'd taken a job at a language school because of its flexible hours;

and at the language school he'd met Abo, now the principal backer of the film.

That was how things happened with Frank.

Abo, intended for a classier seat of learning, was having his troubles with English. Meanwhile, fantastically rich, palatially housed, he wasn't averse to casting a few alms in a direction that guaranteed him a ready supply of boys and girls.

Mooney wondered what had gone wrong there. She had an idea something had. But mainly she wondered about Frank. You could always raise Frank somewhere. She hadn't been able to raise him for two days now.

Something funny was going on.

Frank wasn't just deviant and not just a hop-head. To say he was degenerate was simply to offer an opening remark on his whole fascinating awfulness.

She was aware that Abo was asking if she wanted more whisky. She thanked him and said she didn't, and went home and resumed phoning.

She had a flat close by in the King's Road.

It was opposite the post office.

*

Artie knew he was late when he left the pub but he didn't hurry. He actually slowed. Steve was keeping something from him.

Every time Frank had been mentioned, the subject had been changed. Okay, there was something with Frank; immediately, without question, he had followed Steve's lead. Now Steve was still doing it.

Artie felt one of his rages building up; felt it in his hands, the desire to smash faces, to break things.

He kept talking, though. Steve might still tell him; as if he'd meant to all the time, but that business had to come first.

The business was lousy.

Abo had called at the shop to give Steve the bills back. He said he wouldn't be paying any more. That left them in a great position; a few hundred feet of film stock left, no way of hiring equipment or costumes for the next scenes. They couldn't

40

even see the results of the night-shooting; the labs wouldn't let the stuff out without money.

'What's the least they'd take?' Steve said.

'Two hundred. It's nothing on what we owe. They've been okay.'

'Well, we'll have to get it,' Steve said.

'What is it with Abo?'

'Who knows? We'll settle him, but it takes time.'

'Can't Frank talk to him?' Artie said.

'He'll have to.'

In the pause Artie said, 'Where is Frank?'

'I don't know,' Steve said.

Artie let some moments elapse.

'Why did he come in to see you?' Artie said.

'He bombed out over the girl. I told you.'

'What were you supposed to do about it?'

'Christ, Artie,' Steve said. 'He *flipped*. He came in in a flipped condition. He wanted his hand held. I held it.'

'He was screwing her, wasn't he?'

'You know Frank doesn't screw girls.'

'He does some bloody thing. Where *is* he now?'

'In bed, I suppose. He's low, leave him alone.'

'If he was in bed, Mary would have got at him.'

'So he's somewhere else. What do you want, Artie?'

Artie wanted to yell *To know why you've got him away from the police.* He knew where Frank would be: at the country pad his old portraitist Dad had left him. They'd been there. No phones, hardly any roads. He'd be hiding while he thought what to do. He waited for Steve to say casually he might have a couple of things to do himself that week-end. Then he would pick Steve up and throw him in the road.

Steve didn't say this. He said, 'What did the police want?'

'You know what they wanted,' Artie said. 'They wanted a list of everybody on the location.'

'Did you give them it?'

'Everyone I knew. Frank wasn't there, was he?'

'Oh, Jesus!' Steve said.

They had got to the restaurant now.

41

'Okay,' Artie said. He left Steve and went in right away.

They were all eating duck inside.

Serge said, *'Ah, le poète en personne. La muse est parmi nous.'*

'Que pouvons-nous lui offrir?' Marc said. *'Qu'est-ce qui va inspirer son âme et son palais aujourd'hui?'*

Artie told them all what they could do.

Steve was crossing the Albert Bridge in a cab. He got off at the other side of the river and hurried into the residential hostel.

He wasn't, strictly speaking, entitled to this favoured accommodation, but he'd managed to keep himself listed as a student.

He let himself into his flat and switched on the light. He had left the door locked that led to his bathroom and bedroom and he unlocked it and switched the light on there, too.

Frank stirred unhealthily in the bed.

'Get up now, Frank,' Steve said.

7

'CHRIST. Must you?' Frank said.

He was shielding his eyes from the light.

'Get up,' Steve said, and waited till Frank did.

Frank groped first for his glasses and put them on. Then the long thin length of him articulated out of the bed. He just had his shirt on. He looked awful.

'God,' he said. He had to clutch at the bed.

Steve didn't help him. 'Take a cold shower,' he said.

'Oh, don't be so fucking beastly.'

'Have a wash, then. I'll make coffee.'

He went and did this and presently Frank appeared in a robe.

'Here we are,' Steve said.

Frank shakily sat and sipped the hot, very black coffee. He looked about sixty. He was thirty. Steve alertly watched him.

'How do you feel?' he said.

'Daisy-like. Flower-fresh.'

'Do you want to talk?'

Frank smacked his foul mouth a little. 'Do I?' he said. 'I don't know. What's been happening in the world?'

'Germaine is all over the front pages, and the back pages, and other pages.'

'Well, she made it,' Frank said. 'She wanted to.'

'What did you do to her?'

'I didn't do anything. And stop looking like a lawyer.'

'They say she was strangled, Frank.'

'Oh, God, do they?'

'Yup.' He poured more coffee. 'What happened?'

Frank was assimilating this.

He said dazedly, 'I was in the King's Road. Going to the night shooting. And there was old Germaine, outside The Gold Key. She said she was going to the river.'

'Why?'

'Well, I don't know why,' Frank said pettishly.

'But you went with her.'

'Did I?' Frank said. 'I think I did. Yes. Down those pissy streets. World's End. That's right. That's what we did do.'

'Frank, had you had a fix?' Steve said gloomily.

'What if I had?'

'All right, then what?'

'Then we got there and saw the lights at the other side, the film lights, and I said didn't she want to come and see, and she said she couldn't.'

'Why not?'

'I don't know.'

'So *you* went.'

'Yes.'

'Where?'

Frank looked round the room. 'Oh, God,' he said. 'I wish I wasn't here.'

'When you left Germaine, Frank,' Steve said patiently, 'you went somewhere. You were going to cross the bridge to those lights at the other side. Did you do that?'

'I think,' Frank said slowly, 'I went home. To bed.'

'And in the morning you got up.'

'Well, of course I did. I had a lecture.'

'I don't think you gave it, Frank.'

'No, I wish you'd stop this. Of course I didn't give the fucking lecture. I told *you* that.'

Steve blinked.

'Why didn't you?' he said.

'Are you imbecilic, or what? A kid on the bus had this transistor. I told you. They do news items between the noise. And I suddenly heard Germaine's name and something about the police, so I got off and bought a paper. It was the early one, full of racehorses and greyhounds. But in the stop press it said she'd been drowned. It blew me out of my mind. I suppose I looked a bit funny.'

'That's right, you did,' Steve said. 'Frank, you walked a long way past the art school to come and tell me that.'

Frank looked at him for some moments.

'You don't think I killed her, do you?' he said.

'Do you know if you did, Frank?'

Frank stared even longer.

'Well, I'm going home, for God's sake. Are you mad?' he said.

'Frank, you've been here a couple of days – do you know that? The police are looking for you.'

'Are they?' Frank said. One lank black lock was touching his glasses and his eyes were squinting behind the thick lenses. 'Steve, you surely don't think –'

'I don't know what to think,' Steve said, 'except you need a better story. We've got to go back over every bit of it, see how much you remember.'

Frank drew his robe a bit closer.

'Have you got a drink?' he said.

'Don't have a drink, Frank.' Steve could smell him. He'd left a bottle of Scotch in the room. All gone. 'Have a cigarette,' he said and lit two. 'Okay. The pissy streets and the river and we're sitting watching the lights, right?'

'Well, nearly,' Frank said. 'We're *leaning*, actually. We leaned on the wall.'

'At the wharf.'

'What wharf? We were on the embankment.'

'Those pissy streets go to the wharves,' Steve said. 'You have to turn off to get to the embankment.'

'Did we?' Frank said.

'Can't you remember?'

Frank thought. 'I remember a street,' he said. 'Fairly hideous. Quite long. Awful.'

'With a power station in it? Lots Road?'

'That's right.' Frank was blinking. 'Lots Road. That's what it was. That *is* clever of you, Steve.'

'Frank, don't take offence,' Steve said. 'But Germaine had done a couple of things for you, hadn't she? Did you sort of – fancy anything just then? Have a small gin, if you want.'

He got up and poured Frank one.

Frank sipped the gin. He said thoughtfully, 'No, I didn't. In point of fact, I was feeling bloody awful. It was cold in the flat. I *was* cold. I didn't fancy anything,' he said.

Steve let a silence settle.

'What kind of wall did you lean on?' he said at last.

'The coping. Fantastic view. Nocturne by Whistler.'

'And you just watched a while and then left her.'

'Yes. Well, hang on. She'd already gone.'

'Where?'

'Back the way we came. I think. I don't know. I mean, I was shivering. I was awful, Steve.'

Steve considered a moment. 'Frank,' he said. 'I don't think you were on the embankment. I think you walked down Lots Road to a wharf. That wall you leaned on was at a wharf. You watched the lights from there.'

'Do you think so, Steve?' Frank said uncertainly.

'I do. If you think hard, you'll remember.'

'Wharves,' Frank said. 'Atmospheric, aren't they?'

'Very. Nocturne-ish. Lights across the water.'

'Yes. Traffic was passing though, Steve,' Frank said unhappily.

'Where?'

'In the road just behind us. I don't think it was a wharf. I mean, we could invent one.'

'Are you sure about the traffic?'

'Positive. I'm sure it wasn't a wharf, Steve.'

'Well, thank Christ for that,' Steve said.

'What do you mean?'

'She was killed on a wharf. The police think it was Cremorne Wharf, the farthest from where you were. She was tangled up in some stuff from there. I don't think you killed her, Frank.'

'Well, thanks very much,' Frank said. He was looking at him with dislike.

'We had to know. You're still on the hook, Frank.'

'Well, I'll have another drink,' Frank said.

'No you won't. How did you get home?'

'I caught a cab. On the corner of Beaufort Street, opposite.'

'Would the driver remember you?'

'Well, how would I know that?'

'Did anyone see you when you got in?'

'Did they? I don't know. Yes, they did. That yellow phantom on the ground floor was in the lavatory. She'd ómitted to lock the door. I tried to get in. Some hurly-burly took place with the door. She flashed her fangs at me, from the throne.'

'Oh, well, that's beautiful. Well, it's worth it, Frank.'

'Worth what?' Frank said.

'It's a risk. They haven't got anyone yet. Still, that's what we do. You're volunteering in the morning, Frank. To the police.'

'What are you talking about? Don't be so absurd,' Frank said, with fright.

'Look, you can't stay here. You haven't been at school, or the language place, or the library. You're not at home. Why aren't you at home, incidentally? What do you mean it was cold in the flat?'

'The heating is off. That old phantom is making them change the boiler. She's frightened of fire,' Frank said sulkily.

'Oh, well, fantastic. Frank, you didn't have any fix. What you had was a cold. You were really lousy. You told Germaine that when you were at the river, and she advised you to go home. So you jumped in a cab – police find cab-driver. And went home – interview with old throne person. In the morning you feel so lousy, though, you ask if I'll let you use my fine heated pad.

46

Well, of course I will. Escort you back to it, put you to bed, you're looking so terrible. You haven't heard about old Germaine. When I tell you tonight, you being so improved, your first thought is to go and tell the police what you know. Fault that!' Steve said.

Frank faulted it right away.

'What are you talking about? I never heard such absurdity. Why should I go and give myself up? You know what the police are like!'

'You aren't giving yourself up. You're eliminating yourself. In effect three of you are reporting there in the morning – you, the cab-driver and the lady in the loo.'

'Oh, yes. Great effect. What if they don't remember?'

'It's a risk,' Steve admitted.

8

'WHAT's up with you? Bark!' Georges said in French.

Ah, bark yourself, Artie silently told him. But he barked. *'Encore une bouteille de St Julien '70!'* They were supposed to yell out the wine orders. It made the place sound busy. It was busy, anyway. He'd been run off his feet since he'd gobbled the meal.

They always had the meal together: the patron Georges; the two other waiters, the chef, the under-chef, the washer-up. From the moment he'd finished his coffee he'd been jumping around.

Up and down the stairs from the store-room below, to the bar, to the kitchen, to the main diner, the two side diners. Set the dishes of crudités. Cut up the bread, prepare the biscuits, the cheeses, butter pots, sugar bowls, cruets, mustard.

Then the early guests had started drifting in; candles lit; before he could sort out the fruit bowls.

Non-stop since then.

It was a good small restaurant, French provincial cuisine.

He was an attraction with his Afro and his good French. He was the only one with regular English, anyway.

He didn't mind it. The money was okay for the nights he worked. He could eat there when he wanted. It was suitable in so many ways. But tonight he was in a black rage.

'*Bonsoir, madame, m'sieur. Etes-vous prêts à commander?*'

'I think we'll lay into a steak unless you recommend –'

English.

'Well, the *Canard à la Rouennaise* is really a dream. The chef has excelled himself.'

'Oh, perhaps in that case –'

'*Le St Julien, '70!*' Serge barked, bustling up with it.

'*Pour la table de quatre, là-bas,*' Artie directed him. There was no sommelier, and Georges mainly did it, but when Georges casually sat down and chatted with the regulars, as he now had, Serge got it. That was the way the atmosphere was subtly maintained; waiters running and barking, Georges genially relaxed.

Artie heard his own tongue glibly running, and brooded.

Steve was keeping something back. Some large unsuspected part was being kept back. He tried to control himself, but it was hard.

He wrote the order and took the menus and hustled through to the kitchen. Albert, gaunt, butcher-aproned, was limping about there, working silently and systematically with his cleaver. There was no confusion in the small kitchen. The under-chef worked swiftly with the sauces and with the desserts. The washer-up kept washing up.

Artie gave in the order, and took out two *purées de marrons Mont Blanc* that the under-chef had ready for him, and served them.

'*Ensuite, servez-vous, s'il vous plaît, du café.*'

'*Oui, monsieur.*' And with a single cognac. He knew this pair. Which meant a trot down to the bar for a new bottle.

'*Un cognac pour moi – et pour toi aussi, chérie?*'

'*Non, seulement du café. M'm, quelle merveille cette Crème Chantilly!*'

'Thank you, madame. I knew you'd like it,' Artie said, in English. They liked that; the two languages coming out of the big Afro. They'd joke about it. '*Une fine, monsieur – ça arrive.*'

He sorted out their dinner mints, for the coffee, on his way down to the bar. On his way up, he left the cognac on the banquette and went into the kitchen to see how the canard was doing.

The under-chef was pouring the sauce over the rich stuffed duck, and he waited, and took it, and dodged Marc on his way out.

It went on like this, and he went on brooding.

No, he'd keep things under control now. There was a pattern, and he'd put everything into it; twenty-four hours a day. He'd invested his whole life in their joint conception. He had suppressed too many things – his own directorial ambitions, his poetry – to blow it now. He couldn't do more than he was doing. He had kept nothing back.

Steve was keeping something back. He felt betrayed.

By one o'clock, still on the trot, he felt his head spinning with the cigar smoke and laughter and the smell of food.

The late diners kept at it, coffee and coffee, and one more liqueur and another. He saw Albert jerking his chin at him at the head of the basement stairs, and followed him down, Albert hop-hopping in front of him.

The chef had taken off his butcher-apron and was in his shabby grey jacket. He had his bit of paper with the food order. They gave in the food orders every night on the suppliers' Ansafones. Artie copied the list into English: poultry and meat, fish, dairy stuff, boulangerie, pâtisserie, fruit and vegetables.

'*Relis-le-moi en français*,' Albert said when he'd finished.

Artie read it back.

'*C'est ça*. Okay,' Albert said, and poured himself a cognac at the bar while Artie used the phone there. Tonight, as always, Albert seemed to think he was actually talking to somebody at the other end.

'Tell him his broccoli was solid shit.'

'Okay,' Artie said.

'If that's his broccoli, he can send cabbage.'

Artie told the Ansafone about the broccoli, and Albert took off without a good night.

The staff taxi turned up at half-past one and waited while the restaurant emptied and they did the preliminary clearing.

Through it all, Artie burned with a sense of betrayal.

Okay, he thought, he wouldn't destroy everything because one part was rotten. He would continue, with the help of the crazy Arab or without him; with Steve or without him. Steve had to be used in the way of everything else.

'Okay, *merci les gars, bonne nuit,*' Georges said.

'*Bonne nuit,*' they said.

'*A demain.*'

'*A demain.*'

Tomorrow was Friday when Artie worked again. He worked in the restaurant on Saturday, too. But Sunday was his.

9

'TEDDY, it's a beautiful day. Why don't you go out there for an hour or two, it will do you good, lift up your spirits,' Mrs Warton said.

She said it without much conviction. From the sullen look on his face something like an exorcist would be needed to get anything going with him in the spirit-raising line. He had all the Sunday papers round him on the bed.

She'd known it wasn't going to be easy when she'd opened the front door, first thing. The sun had glinted into the porch and on to the fat wad of papers lying there. It had glinted on a section of Ted's nose which disappeared over the fold of the top one. The headline bore the word Chelsea. A quick flip revealed the same word in all the headlines.

'Have they come yet?' he had bawled from upstairs.

'Yes, dear, bringing them right up.'

Oh, dear. Ted *would* be upset, she had thought. And Ted was.

'Don't bother having a shave,' she coaxed him now. Shaving was dangerous. He thought while shaving. 'Just jump into your togs and get me a few sprouts, and something for the vases. My word, the air is like wine, do you a world of good.'

Without a word, with something more in the nature of a hawk or belch, Warton swept the papers on the floor and thrust a foot out of bed.

He had quite a decent morning in the garden, however; got the old runner beans down and on the compost heap, poles stacked in the shed. There was a bit of slug about; all the damp weather. He'd do for them next week. Wallflowers getting a bit stalky in the boxes; should be planted out, really. No time before lunch.

He became aware something hadn't happened. Rose hadn't come out to ask him if he wanted to slip up the road for one before lunch. Well, he didn't. Catch him showing his face in there today. She was thoughtful, Rose.

His heart lurched again, all the same.

Need a bloody miracle to save him now.

Oh yes, it was all happening, artists' studies of Germaine in the altogether. Reporters buzzing round that art school like blue-arsed flies. His own little outburst when he'd told them to stop hounding him and to go to the Information Room at the Yard. ('Take the pressure off you, Ted,' the C.C. had said. Warton had been going to ask to be relieved of Press conferences, but it had thrown him into a stupor. Why had it been suggested to him first?)

And the little hints and nudges in the papers; three apparently motiveless murders in a fortnight within a mile of each other. They'd used different words for the same menacing suggestion ... 'Inquiries being made at mental institutions for inmates who ...'

Oh yes, oh yes.

'Lunch, dear.'

Thoughtful, Rose.

The kids weren't here this week-end.

Very thoughtful.

Why was she being so thoughtful? Why everybody so thoughtful? Take the pressure off. Nice relaxing week-end. Needed relaxing, did he?

Warton snouted through his roast beef and sprouts and York-shire pud.

Didn't give any hint, though. Not his way. Ng. Ur.

He didn't do much really, just waited for tomorrow's papers. Put another hour in, in the garden, but no heart for it. He sat sullenly watching the box all evening, and went to bed early.

He slept badly and woke to catch only the tail end of the radio news. Earthquake, had the chap said?

He shot down to pick up the papers himself.

Earthquake. South America. Huge devastation.

Well, well.

He had a bath and a shave and watched himself carefully in the mirror.

Not a bad moment to feed them the pregnancy. Drop it in and let them figure it out; in and around earthquake specials. Showed a line being pursued. Useful. Right moment.

'Shocking news, Teddy,' Rose said, shovelling him his eggs.

'Terrible. Quite a few thousand dead, I see.'

Yes, and a nice wave of typhus, if he knew anything about it. Hundreds of thousands homeless. Special appeals, Red Cross, Pope, blankets. Keep them all busy.

'Those poor souls.'

'Shocking.' He went out to the car with something like spring in his heel. Weather holding up. Very promising day.

'Right. Everybody here?' he said in his office when the team had assembled.

'All in, sir. Shut the door, last man,' Summers said.

'I just want to say that now we no longer have to worry about Press briefings, I intend instituting fuller conferences between ourselves. I see one or two new faces today,' he said, looking round at the thirty-odd detectives. 'Soon get the routine next door. Don't want to go into it now.' Next door was the Incident Room, where a most formidable routine had been established; by him.

'Just one word, subject of the Press, before we leave it. Very useful organ, the Press. Operative word, useful. To us. Don't want it vice-versa. Our duty, pursue our investigations thoroughly, without deflection. However, deflection sometimes unavoidable.

'What we have here, three unconnected murders. Press wants a connection. No lead turns up, they dream one. Doing it now – you'll have seen. Round-up of nut-houses, likely nutters on parole. Very irresponsible. So – deflection needed.

'This morning, Information Room at the Yard will be putting out a piece of evidence we'd sooner have kept. Germaine Roberts was in the tenth week of pregnancy. Forensically very important. However, give a dog a bone. Lesser of two evils.

'Next point. Most important, investigation of this kind, keep an open mind. Press is working up to a maniac. All right, maybe there *is* one. Can't rule it out. Am therefore instituting from today what I call the Crazy Ideas department. Note the word. Not unorthodox. Crazy. Don't want anybody to think he's a fool. Any man with an idea – bring it to Chief Inspector Summers, or to me. Won't laugh. Assure you of that. Contrary. Those who know me know I'm not a big laugher.'

He heard quiet appreciation of that one round the room. No harm in dropping in a comical touch from time to time. Didn't look up or acknowledge it in any way. Not a bloody comedian.

He listened expressionlessly as Summers read out the Cumulative. The landlord Logan had been ruled out; timing didn't allow his involvement on a wharf. Dr Frank Colbert-Greer had been interrogated and his story checked. Investigations were proceeding with a gay club, Shaft, adjacent to Cremorne Wharf; Germaine Roberts had been a member.

'Right,' Summers said, winding up. 'All those whose assignments aren't ready, go to the waiting room or hop down to the canteen. There's too much hullabaloo in that Incident Room. Caught me on the hop a bit, this briefing, sir,' he apologized to Warton.

'Ng,' Warton said in absolution. Not a big brain, Summers. Could organize, though. 'How was it?' he said, when they'd all shuffled out.

'Put heart into them, sir.' Summers filled his pipe, nodding sincerely. '*Esprit de corps*,' he said over the flame of his match.

'Ng,' Warton said, pleased. 'Which one Mason?'

Summers had mentioned the young detective he considered promising.

'Tall lad, cleft chin, longish hair.'

'Long hair, eh?'

'Protective colouring. Ambitious lad,' said Summers.

*

The ambitious lad had tabbed follow-ups in Bywater Street; known as 'sit-downs'. He had no objection. He did his work, noted those needing still further inquiry, and was through before one.

He had a pint and a sandwich at the Markham Arms, and took a small trundle along nearby Jubilee Place, scene of Miss Manningham-Worsley's exit.

Very weird, the murders so close together.

He thought he'd have a look at the area of the third, down by the river.

The King's Road was busy at lunch-time, a coppery sun glinting. He bought a paper; front page full of the earthquake. Big scratchy wire photo of a woman in a bowler hat crying with a child in her arms. Relief supplies being sent, message from the Pope, blankets. A little teaser at the foot of the page said *Chelsea Model was Pregnant, page 5*.

Page 5, eh? Not bad thinking, Ng, he thought.

He picked his way across the road and went down Flood Street. Plumply prosperous houses, done up to the knocker. There was a copper outside Mrs Thatcher's, but nothing special in that: important politician.

He cut through to Cheyne Walk.

Well, this was the life, Mason thought. He was a Battersea lad himself, brought up on the opposite bank of the river. He'd always admired the discreet splendour of the pads on this side. He strolled past the huge gated mansions of Cheyne Walk set back, behind trees, from the hazy flowing river.

Henry VIII's old estate, as he knew from school. Elizabeth I brought up here. All private houses now, of course. Marvellous brick, clad in creepers, lightly pock-marked with plaques to other illustrious residents.

He paused at one and read the inscription. George Eliot, novelist.

He strolled on, reading the others. Dante Gabriel Rossetti, Algernon Charles Swinburne.

Well, well, all the lads.

In the pleasant sun, filtered through trees and falling leaves, Mason walked on, spelling out the plaques until Cheyne Walk ended and he was out on the roaring embankment, traffic thundering past.

He watched for an opportunity to cross the road, and found it, close by a testimonial to another famous resident. James McNeill Whistler, painter. Appropriate enough : the river began its sharp turn into Whistler's Reach at that point.

Mason wove through the lines of huge container trucks and hit the opposite pavement, and found the position where Colbert-Greer had stood with the girl and stood there himself. He leaned on the stone coping and looked across the Thames.

From here the abandoned wharf where they'd been filming was plainly visible. To his right, along Whistler's Reach, the industrial skyscape, Lots Road power station. All added up.

Weird guy, Greer. Mason hadn't seen him but he'd heard from the Cumulative of the follow-ups. Cab-driver checked out, old woman in the toilet checked out. She'd apparently had her transistor in there with her; listening to the end of a radio play, which timed it. He was apparently in the clear. Apparently.

Mason mused, looking about him, hands on the sun-warmed coping. He tried to imagine it the other night; a chilly night. Greer shivering, unsteady on his feet. (Independent reports of that; tall thin geezer seen with girl on the embankment, swaying. The girl had left first; independent reports of that, too.)

Had he followed her? Could he have done?

Not in the time, he couldn't; not all the way to Cremorne Wharf and back. Why would he have come back, anyway? He could have cut through to the King's Road from there.

But the cabbie had picked him up here; just opposite, on the corner of Beaufort Street. Mason turned and looked there. The driver had seen Greer waving at him as he swayed across the road, pointing in the direction of Beaufort Street; had pulled round the corner and waited for him there. In Greer had popped, and off they'd immediately gone, to the other end of the New King's Road.

No, Greer had been safely home while Gabriel was still walking to her fate.

There was something wrong with that. It took a moment to see what it was. Not Gabriel. *Germaine*. Diane *Germaine* Roberts. The other name had put him off. It took a while longer to remember the other name and where he'd seen it. Rossetti. Dante Gabriel Rossetti. Same initials.

Something stirred in his mind, another formulation of initials. Close by Dante Gabriel Rossetti had been Algernon Charles Swinburne. Familiar that. Why?

The subject of his recent sit-downs surfaced.

Alvin C. Schuster.

A.C.S. . . . D.G.R. Funny.

He tried to think of the other one, the old lady. Manningham-Worsley. What was her first name . . .? Jane. J.M.W. Anything there?

He frowned along Whistler's Reach, trying to think what might be there, until with slow dawning came the name of the patron of the Reach. It was James McNeill Whistler's Reach.

Well, Jesus, Mason thought.

Well, hang on, he thought.

People had to have *some* initials. You could get almost anything out of initials. Look at old Algernon out of a simple A. Or old Alvin, come to that.

He wondered if he should double back and look at all the plaques again to see how many had similar initials. But Chelsea was full of plaques. There must be a list somewhere.

He saw a number 49 bowling over Battersea Bridge and ran for it. The lights were at red but they changed just as he made it.

'Right for King's Road?' he called.

'Hop on, mate,' the conductor said.

He hopped on. 'Where's the library there?' he said.

'Manresa Road, five pence.'

Mason made inquiry at the central counter and was directed

upstairs to the reference library. He went up the two flights, pushed the swing doors and entered a rather oppressive silence.

People were scattered about the large room, sitting at mahogany desks. There was no one at the counter, so he looked around and presently espied a girl stacking books on shelves on a gallery at the far end. He gave her a cough and she turned and motioned that she'd be down. She came immediately.

Oh, yes. Very nice little bird, Mason thought. Victorian looking, yellow hair, parted in the middle; something a bit classical happened to it at the back.

'I was wondering if you had a list of plaques,' he said.

'Plaques?'

'A list of the famous people who have –'

'Oh, yes. We have. Would you like to come upstairs with me?'

Not half, Mason thought. He followed her behind the counter, through a door, up a steep flight of stairs. Not bad legs; hips a bit plump. All the sweeter. Very refined little thing; quick, neat, clean. Oh yes; have a helping there, any time.

She led him to a stuffy attic, crammed with books. It was dark and she put the light on.

'This section is local records,' she said. Shelves filled with booklets, pamphlets, parish magazines. She fingered neatly through. 'Here we are. Would you like to see it here?'

'Thanks.'

She left him and Mason sat and studied the list. It was a three-pager, duplicated, in a cover. It took him only one look through to see that nobody else had the same initials as the three sets he'd got. Astounded, slightly stunned, he went through it again.

No. Just those.

Well, damn it, he thought.

He took the list and went below.

'Can I borrow this?' he said.

'Sorry. Nothing can be taken from the reference library.'

'Well.' He had to have it. 'I noticed a copier below. Can I just go and copy it?'

'Nothing's allowed to leave this room.'

'I'd leave you my driving licence,' Mason said, smiling.

'Sorry . . .'

Jesus. He'd have to show her. He took his wallet out and withdrew enough of his warrant card for her to see. The girl's eyes went curiously over him.

'Go on, I'll only be a tick,' Mason said, wrinkling his nose as he smiled, which he knew often worked.

'Be ever so quick, then.'

Mason was quick. Five minutes later he was out in Manresa Road again, with the copy, his heart thudding.

Two things had occurred to him. One was that whatever the significance of his find, it couldn't fail to do him a power of good. Scotland Yard and Fleet Street combined had so far failed to discover a single connecting factor between the murders.

He had just gone and discovered one.

It could rocket a young cop up through the firmament.

The other thing was that he might have a dab at the pussy cat in the reference library. She'd told him her name: Brenda. She was interested in him, he could see that.

First things first, though.

10

MASON was right about the pussy cat, but for the wrong reasons. Brenda was interested. She hated sitting like a dummy all night with the clever talk going on round her. Sometimes they had the actors and actresses, which she much preferred. She knew she was prettier than a lot of the girls, but they had more to say. She was flattered they asked her, really.

She had been asked to The Potters for that night, so she was glad she had something to say.

The only thing was, Frank was there, and he made her sick.

'Did he fancy you, darling?' Frank said, nodding at her. 'You know, sniff-sniff. Did he go sniff-sniff?'

'I don't know, I'm sure,' Brenda said.

'Bet he did. Take my word for it. I've developed a taste for detectives. I feel a frisson when one is near.'

Something had happened to Frank, they'd all noticed it. Steve had told him to wrap up a couple of times, and she wished he would. He made her physically ill.

'Why a list of plaques?' Steve said.

'It isn't just plaques. It's all the famous residents – all the dead ones, Sir Thomas More and Thomas Carlyle. It's partly the Greater London Council list, you know, G.L.C., and partly –'

'What did he want with it?' Steve said.

She wished she could say *'Darling, I don't know,'* like the actresses. She couldn't make herself form the words, despite the two gin-and-tonics she'd had. She wished some other girls would show up. She felt exposed with the three men.

'Isn't Mary Mooney coming?' she said.

'Mooney-Mooney-we-won't-tell-Mooney,' Frank chanted.

Steve looked at him. 'Why not?' he said.

'We won't,' Frank said, with a little nod. 'That's all.' He kept nodding, and also twirling a little string of worry beads that he had lately taken to carrying.

Brenda felt her head going round with the beads, and the gin-and-tonics. She picked up her handbag. 'Excuse me a moment,' she said, and headed for the Ladies'.

'What are you thinking of?' Steve said.

'We could have fun,' Frank said.

'How?'

'I don't know. I'll think. I will have a little chat with *Brendah,*' Frank said, camping up the name. 'Tell her to forget it.'

'Yeah, she's bound to from you,' Artie said.

Frank looked at him with dislike. 'Why are you being such a beast this evening?'

'Oh, bugger off,' Artie told him.

'Well, thank you, fans.'

Steve was watching Artie. He was certainly bugged. Steve knew what was bugging him, and he thought it childish. He'd already privately explained why he hadn't been able to tell him about Frank until the matter was straightened out.

'I will have a chat with Brendah,' Frank said again.

'No, skip it,' Steve said. He could see this was bugging Artie,

59

too. Everything was bugging him lately. Anyway, he knew the girl would forget the matter if nobody said anything. He saw Brenda appearing, distantly, and got up himself. 'I've had enough for one night,' he said.

'So soon?' Frank said. 'What's up with everyone? What you all need is a session with the detectives. They perk a fellow up. In fact, *everything* needs perking up. Isn't that right, darling?' he said, as Brenda, rather pale, stood beside them.

'What?' Brenda said, despite herself.

But playful Frank wouldn't tell her. He just twirled his beads as they left the pub. That was lateish on Monday night.

*

The envelope arrived on Wednesday. Because it was addressed just to *Murder HQ, Chelsea Police Station*, it went first to the clerks in the Incident Room. It was a long white envelope, and inside was a sheet of cartridge paper folded in three.

On the sheet were four lines of Letraset Gothic lettering, carefully placed. They read:

> She had three lilies
>   in her hand
> And the stars in her hair
>   were seven.

There was nothing else in the envelope, so the clerk who had opened it simply recorded its arrival in the Journal, with the day and the time, Wednesday, 2.30 p.m.; which marked the official start of the Chelsea Murders (Series II).

Two

To dance to flutes,
  To dance to lutes,
Is delicate
  And rare.

11

Two miles up the road, Mooney was in her customary position for the day and the hour. The day was the same Wednesday, the hour ten. She was looking along her jeans-clad legs, stretched on the next chair, and nodding glumly at what was coming at her out of the phone.

Taking one with another, Wednesdays were bloody terrible. Everything started again on Wednesday. It was like Sisyphus rolling his stone to the top of the hill and never getting there. Something of an anti-climactic nature did actually happen here once a week, but it happened on Tuesday. The last pages went off to Dorking then, for printing on Wednesday, publication dated Friday.

The *Gazette* was one of a chain of eight suburban papers sharing common advertising and features. Their own news pages had to be dovetailed in with the others, which meant the least newsworthy items had to go first; hence the regular Wednesday dredge of municipal offices, churches, clubs.

Not Fleet Street.

'Well, I'm sure everyone realizes that, Monty,' she said.

She was talking to Montague Humboldt of the Artists' Guild. He was giving her an earful about the national disgrace of Normanby's widow being on public assistance.

'They don't, Mary, honestly!' Monty said, excitedly.

He continued raving so she cast an eye over the proof pages. VICAR RAPS CHURCH VANDALS. *'Beastliness' in Vestry*. Not bad, but it had only made page 7; he hadn't specified the beastliness even to Len Offard, who had done the story.

Len was sitting opposite her now, at the other side of the twin banks of ancient roll-top desks. He was using his own phone, and she was distracted by the need to keep an ear open for what he was saying. He wasn't discussing the *Gazette*'s business, but his own; he was talking to *The Sun*. She was almost sure it was about the murders because of the extreme abbreviation of his remarks and the way his eyes flitted shiftily over hers.

Old Monty kept going.

'. . . think the G.L.C. at least would have the grace to mark in some way the studio where he created his greatest . . .'

'I thought they had, Monty.'

'Of course you did. People do think that,' Monty said. 'Yet not so much as a –'

Mooney made a note. Might be something. Nothing on the public assistance issue. Normanby's widow hadn't suffered in silence. Marking of studios, though : G.L.C. falling down on the job.

'Where was his studio – Tite Street?'

'No. You see ! Glebe Place. Near where Galsworthy wrote –'

Galsworthy, eh? Not bad. 'Okay, Monty, I'll look into it. Are you sure he's not listed anywhere?'

'Oh, *listed* possibly,' Monty said contemptuously, 'but I can assure you –'

'Lovely. 'Bye, Monty.' She hung up and jiggled the phone. 'Sandra, can you put me through to Wilfred.'

'He's right here, Mary.'

Yes, course he was.

'Yes, Mary?'

'Wilfred, I want something on Stanley Normanby. Is his old studio listed anywhere?'

'Normanby. I'll call you.'

As Mooney hung up, two things struck her. One was that Len had hung up at the identical moment with a very smug look on his face. The other was the old pub slate with messages, hung on the wall. Someone had chalked on it MOONEY IS SPOONY. This could only be a reference to Otto Wertmuller. She had done a diary item on him, describing his scrumptiousness in perhaps extravagant terms.

She brooded on this as she tidied the items collected so far.

Wertmuller had been blond and gorgeous and gentle, despite his build, which was along cave-man lines. He had that kind of hair that needed fingers running through it. She had felt a slight itch in her fingers at sight of it. His own fingers had been beautiful, long and delicate and capable of all sorts of useful stuff on their own account.

Mooney put together a small item from the Citizens' Advice Bureau, relevant to unmarried mothers, still brooding. Wertmuller hadn't evidently felt the need for an immediate grab at her; no calls, no follow-ups, though she'd been particularly careful to give him both numbers, office and home.

What the devil was going on of late?

Mooney was no hysterical advocate of the need for the body's rapture, but she thought fair was fair, and that people ought to get their share. Of latter months she had been wondering what had happened to hers. This thing and that had fallen through to her considerable bemusement. She got around, saw people, chatted. Month after raptureless month had withered away.

She had a quick look along the length of herself, and felt a compulsive need for a look at her face, too, so she got out her compact and had one.

'It's Len, old chap,' Len said on the phone, opposite her, carefully not mentioning the old chap's name. 'Anything doing?'

It was looking a bit old, her face, leathery, experienced. But as faces went, it was full of character, intelligent, amusing, falling easily into a smile. She let it fall into one to see what it looked like. It looked fine. It had laughed its head off, had that face, for the benefit of likely-looking rapturists.

Her phone rang.

'News room,' she said.

'You've got that list,' Wilfred said.

'*I* have?'

'Your initials here, M.M.'

She *had* had the list – a little story about Augustus John, three weeks ago – but it had gone back. She was certain of it. He had come and taken it back himself.

'It isn't here now,' she said.

'Well, you're not signed out.'

Of course she wasn't signed out. He'd *taken* it. Probably gone down and hung around Sandra at the switchboard. He'd got it filed under something else by now, mind full of rapture.

'Aren't there any other copies about?' she said.

'At Manresa Road. How about this one, though?'

'Well, I haven't got it, Wilfred. I haven't sold it.'

'Your initials, you see.'

'Yeah, okay, Wilfred.'

Silly little clot.

All the silly little clots were getting their rapture.

Everyone in the world was.

It wasn't making her sour. She had a quick look at her face to see that it wasn't. She saw vestigial expressions there – one of faint scorn had just crossed it – that Wertmuller had not had the benefit of. She was almost certain he hadn't, and it was rather good. She tried it again. She saw Len watching her, and examined her teeth instead.

'Many thanks, old chap,' Len said. 'Much appreciate it.'

He hung up and went out.

Mooney closed her compact, torn between thoughts of Wertmuller's fingers and the public neglect of Normanby and the chap who had just earned Len's appreciation.

She picked up her phone and called the *Globe*.

'Chris? Mooney here. Anything doing?'

'Hello, Mary.' He immediately began talking to someone in the office without even asking her to hang on. Her heart slowly sank. What *was* it with everything lately? She'd got them a marvellous exclusive. It was practically her story. Was this getting away from her, too? And just because she'd fallen down on a couple of things, Frank and the pregnancy. She'd been certain a few days ago that they would offer her a job. Certain of it . . .

'Mary, I'm tied up now. Is it anything special?'

'No, I was only wondering –'

'Okay, we'll call if we need anything.'

'All right,' Mooney said quietly, and hung up and sat with her stomach turned to lead.

She thought that the best thing would be to go home and have a bath and get back in bed with the covers over her head.

Then she thought, no it wouldn't. What with the general

maladjustment of things, she was going to have a treat. She was going to have a look at Wertmuller; a huge ample thing, top to toe and back again. While at it – he was only across the way from Manresa Road – she would look into the library and see what could be done about poor neglected Normanby.

Neglect, neglect. People could die of it, even the dead.

*

She didn't know what she'd say to Wertmuller, but as it happened she didn't have to say anything. She walked through to the backroom of Options & Renewals (the option was of selling them stuff or getting them to repair it) and he just rose from his chair, foot after foot of him, with the most glorious smile ever seen on human face.

'Mary,' he said, 'oh, Mary, it is so nice to see you.'

'H-h-hello, Otto. I – I –'

'I had no means of getting in touch. I am late last night back from Germany. My father was seriously ill.'

'Oh. Was he? I mean is he –'

'Now, thank God, he is recovered. But all the time, Mary, I thought of you.'

Oh, well, damn it, Mooney thought. She didn't know whether to pick a square metre of him and start in kissing or simply pass out on the floor from sheer gratitude. He had a sort of viola in his arms and he put it down and took her hands.

'You have walked in as if to my dream,' he said.

Was she hearing aright? She didn't want to shake her head and clear it because it was fine the way it was. If it was a dream, this was the kind to have.

'Just now I sat and wondered what you must think of me, if perhaps I have queered my – boats?'

'Pitch,' Mooney said. God! No. You haven't, Otto. All yours, the whole pitch.

She wasn't rightly certain what else he said. In conjunction with that fantastic twinkle in his eye, slightly triste, absolutely bang-on, and his hair, and his whole God-sent self, he was gently kneading her hands with those unbelievable fingers. What was needed was some kind of computer to store, to bank, and then feed back moment after golden moment of it for all her remaining years.

She didn't know if it was rash or not, she just damn well invited him to dinner. She wrapped it up somehow, didn't know what friends he'd made as yet . . . She was only passing, on Press business – And how was that frame that had so interested her?

He gladly showed her the frame. He had this notion – the newly opened shop had called the paper two or three weeks ago, to milk a bit of publicity – that old picture frames were often finer works of art than those they enclosed. He restored them, and old things generally. He was a very good restorer.

Oh, boy, and how! Mooney thought, running recklessly across the road towards the library and the restoration of Normanby's reputation.

Righto, Normanby! she said to herself. After what you've done for me, you've got something coming. I'll see you right, Normanby. I'll take on the G.L.C., the Government, the U.N., Idi Amin. It's you and me, Normanby!

She raced up the two flights like a mountain goat.

'My word, Brenda – your hair!'

She hadn't seen the girl lately.

'Don't you like it?' Brenda said, nervously touching it.

'Like it? It's fantastic.'

'Is it? Only nobody's said anything.'

'Smashing, love. It transforms you.'

'Oh, well,' Brenda said, transformed, and just stood and breathed for a moment. 'And I'm going out with a chap tonight,' she said.

Mooney well understood that this girl's basic life urge at the moment was to lay hands on a mirror, but she sped on. 'I want the listing of Normanby's old studio – the artist. You've got it here somewhere, haven't you?'

'Yes. In Special Collections. You know where it is.'

'Don't know if I can find it. Is Frank up there?'

'Not yet. I'll show you, then. That's funny,' Brenda said, leading the way. 'You're the second this week for that list. We had a detective in here.'

'Oh, yes.'

Brenda was so sent by her hair she forgot for a moment that somebody had said Mooney wasn't to know. Then she remembered it was Frank who'd said it, and she had a rude thought about Frank.

Mooney was so sent by Wertmuller that she didn't all at once take in what had been said.

When she did, and between proffering her compact and the odd word on hair, she unravelled what had gone on.

Later, alone with the list, she sat and quietly marvelled at how things went, when they went for you.

She thought of heavenly Otto and the job on the *Globe*, both, less than an hour ago, apparently lost to her.

She stationed Wertmuller in a portion of her mind convenient for later attention, and bent to the list.

It took only a few lightning swings round the battlefield to see where the panzers had to go in.

When she left the library she had the dope on Normanby and some other dope.

One of the troubles with the *Globe*, she thought, was that they didn't know how to treat a girl right. Call her when needed, would they? There were other fish in the sea. She knew how a certain percentage of them, in the region of a hundred per cent, would react to what she had to offer.

Pow!

She had no intention of offering yet. Certain subjects needed a little coaxing; subjects like Wertmuller came in this class.

Mooney made a couple of purchases at nearby shops and sprang lithely up to her flat opposite the post office before resuming serious work.

That was at about eleven.

12

Soon after half-past two, when the envelope and its contents went in to Warton, he lost himself in a cloud of smoke and brooded. His standing instructions in any major inquiry were that all letters for his HQ should be delivered immediately by special messenger from local post offices, and this one had been.

It had been mailed at the main post office in the King's Road. It had slipped down the chute from the external box some time between 1 p.m. and 2 p.m., but because it was the lunch hour, and staff short, the exact time couldn't be established.

He had the material copied and the originals sent for specialist examination, and by three o'clock had dispatched Mason to the library.

Mason was driven round in solitary grandeur, and mounted right away to the second floor.

'If I wanted to look up some lines of a poem,' he said to the bird, 'how would I go about it?'

'Have you got the poet's name?'

'No.'

'Oh. Over here, then.' She took him to Dictionaries and pointed out the volumes of quotations.

'What's the poem about?' she said.

'Suppose it was the moon.'

She took down an *Oxford*. 'Well, you just look up this index at the back,' she said, 'and there you are. Moon.'

'Thanks,' Mason said.

He waited till she'd gone and looked up lilies.

A close-packed column on lilies.

Lilies.

> *Beauty lives though l. die.*   208:9.

He went down the column.

> *Three l. in her hand.*   410:7.

He turned to page 410, quotation 7.

> The blessed damozel leaned out
> From the gold bar of heaven;
> Her eyes were deeper than the depth
> Of waters stilled at even;
> She had three lilies in her hand,
> And the stars in her hair were seven.

The name of the poem was 'The Blessed Damozel', and the poet Dante Gabriel Rossetti.

Mason copied all this, replaced the book, and took off.

*

By half-past three Warton was snouting through 'The Blessed Damozel'.

'Gold bar, sir,' Summers said.

'Ng.'

'Waters stilled at even.'

'Well aware of it, Summers.' He thought if Summers kept pointing out possible allusions to The Gold Key and the nocturnal Thames, he'd do for him.

Some clever bastard was having them on here. Some clever *literary* bastard. The message, envelope, type, cartridge paper, were still with the experts; nothing at all to feed on except his own yellow rage.

'Any further thoughts, Mason?' he said.

They'd already been through it. The lad swore he'd told nobody. Bloody obvious his idea had got out somewhere. Warton had spotted the loophole himself, and waited for the lad to spot it. He knew Summers wouldn't. Summers didn't. Lad did.

'Well, it *could* have got out through the library, sir.'

'How?'

'The girl saw my warrant card. Though I only asked for the list, sir.'

'Who could gather anything from that?'

'Perhaps – this fellow Colbert-Greer?' Mason said slowly.

'How?'

'Well, he might have been reading about these murders, and if she mentioned a detective had asked for the list – could have looked at it himself, made the same connection. He was working there, after all. So was this coloured bloke, the one interested in police records.'

'Were they there when you were?'

'No.'

'What do you think, then?'

Saw him make the next leap. 'Well, if they were regulars, the girl might have had friendly relations with them.'

'Think she has?'

'Worth looking into, sir.'

Yes. He'd do.

'Go to it,' Warton said.

*

Summers and Mason saw the chief librarian together in his small office. After a preliminary chat, Brenda was called in.

It was twenty-to five by this time, and she'd just been to the rest room to give her hair a touch. The library closed at five on Wednesdays, and she was meeting the chap at Sloane Square at quarter-past.

'These gentlemen are from the police, Brenda,' the librarian said. 'They'd like to ask you a few questions.'

She saw Mason nodding at her, and her heart turned over. She thought immediately of Frank and his horrid sniff-sniff remarks, and she knew it was to do with him.

'Oh, yes?' she said.

'Sit down, dear.'

She sat down, a bit wobbly.

She'd actually planned to get off a bit early. Didn't want to keep the chap waiting. First time she'd been out with him.

'I expect you remember Mr Mason here.' It was the tall gaunt one talking. 'Came in first a couple of days ago.'

'Yes.'

'Do you remember what he wanted then?'

'A list of plaques, wasn't it, of famous residents?'

Mason just nodded at her; didn't say anything.

'Did you mention that to anyone?'

'I *might* have done,' she said.

'It's rather important,' the gaunt one said. 'There wouldn't be anything wrong in it, no reason why you shouldn't.'

'Well.' She made a pretence of thinking. All she could think of was horrible Frank, twirling his beads.

Bit by bit, she let it slip out, keeping it quite ladylike. The chief librarian wouldn't think she was *getting off* with the readers, would he? Thank God, he was nodding approvingly at her. The others just watched and listened. They made her go over it again and again: who'd been in the pub circle; what talk there had been about the list, what questions asked.

She saw that it was two minutes to five, and then, oh God, two minutes after, and they were still going on. She didn't like to mention her date, not after this particular pub date.

'And that's absolutely all that happened?'

'Oh, yes.'

Five-past five. And she absolutely had to have a wee after all this.

'And you didn't mention it to anyone else?'

'Oh, no.'

'Well, I think that's about all. I'd be glad if you wouldn't mention it elsewhere for the time being.'

'Oh, you won't do that, Brenda, will you?' the chief librarian said.

'Oh, no!' Brenda said, renouncing all sin.

'Well, thank you, dear.'

She hared off to the loo, made short work of that, grabbed her bag and coat and was in the King's Road like a jet. God above, it was nearly quarter-past! Taxi fare was a lunch, but she saw an empty one and threw herself in. 'Sloane Square!'

In the cab she had a quick look at her face and licked up her lipstick and gave her hair a bit of a touch. In the same moment she remembered that she *had* told someone else.

Well, damn it, they weren't interested in Mary, and if they were – twenty-past five! – they could jolly well go and do something a bit rude.

*

There had been several sets of fingerprints on the envelope –

73

which Warton knew would lead nowhere at all – but none on the cartridge paper. The paper-makers hadn't yet been identified, but the Letraset people were compiling a list of customers who had taken the rather unusual type style. In general, it was used by advertising agencies, graphics studios and art schools. But more information would come from the wholesale stationers, whom they also supplied, and who in turn supplied shops selling artists' materials, several of which were in the King's Road.

The list of Famous Residents had apparently been circulated in an edition of fifty copies. Warton skipped the various civic authorities who had it, and concentrated on those with public access. There were not very many.

He wrote out the general assignment, and sent it through to Summers. As head of the Incident Room, it was Summers's job to break it down and allot the work.

After this, and in an unusual mood of good cheer, Warton thought he would have an early night. In the hellish reaches of the afternoon, an amazingly good idea had come to him.

He thought he'd keep the idea to himself for the time being.

He gave a gruff 'G'night' to the Incident Room and took himself off.

He could see the scenario of his idea in its tiniest portions, and all of it looked good. Apart from the scenario, he could also see his plate, so lately piled high with mountains of unlooked-for crap.

Long years at his job had made Warton familiar with its unpleasant patterns. All the way to Sanderstead he visualized the extra crap now undoubtedly being created for him by the spry and imaginative chefs of Fleet Street.

Yes, best of luck, Warton wished them, turning cheerfully into his drive.

13

'By way of starters,' Jack said, 'I'd like to spring this on Friday. Nothing doing on Saturday. Then depending on how the Sundays play it – number two. For Monday, perhaps Tuesday.'

Number two was headed THE SIEGE OF CHELSEA. The two men were studying roughs in the editor's office. Jack was secretive about the roughs. He'd taken them out of a drawer after the editorial conference was over and the other departmental heads had left.

It was now Thursday and they were through with the earthquake. A few hundred were being added daily to the death toll but there was no excitement in the streets on the latest score.

Next week was national maniac week; it was obvious.

'What basically worries me,' Chris said, 'is not to blow it too early.'

'Which?'

'The Siege.'

'Yes. It's a beaut, isn't it?' Jack said.

A pencil-sketched policeman stood all down the left-hand side of the page; evidently in an alley in lamplight. His helmet was turned steadfastly towards the huge headline. Above it, a two-line strap outlined the gravity of what he was watching.

'Wednesday or Thursday,' Jack mused, 'would definitely be better. Allow the story to build. Too risky, though. It's our siege at the moment. Which means playing this one rather close.'

He was tapping number one. This one just said SCOTLAND YARD BAFFLED. There were four photos; three of the recent dead, and a larger one of the man looking into the deaths.

'It's the nutter theory, is it?' Chris said anxiously.

'Oh, yes. Great piece from the shrink, by the way. We'll need plenty of supporting ideas.'

'Yes. The snag there,' Chris said, 'is that there aren't any. No actual hard stuff, you see, Jack.'

'That definitely isn't our fault. If they're not putting it out, we'll make them. If they haven't got it, why haven't they?'

'Well, true, but –'

'I mean, what are we expressing but the general anxiety people must be feeling? If the Yard is worried – Christ, so am I. I as reader. I mean, what's happening? Plenty to go for, surely?'

'Well, there's no doubt –'

'Panic stalking the streets being the staple. In which connection – Violet's piece. Far too chatty. All these people carrying on as usual. They shouldn't be carrying on as usual. We need some genuine nervousness. Cinema takings *down* – locksmiths' takings *up*. What time are they bolting in the old folks? Things of that nature. We can take your other ideas now.'

They discussed Chris's other ideas, but he was by no means at ease with them. 'What would make me happier, Jack, is some *hard* stuff. This film group Mooney was keen on. She seemed to think –'

'Oh, God, she isn't still going on about it, is she?'

'Not at all. I can't even raise her. But there's apparently an Arab backing the film.'

'You're not suggesting he's backing the maniac?'

'No.'

'Then change gear,' the editor advised. 'This thing is big.'

'Okay,' Chris said.

'As are Arabs in season. But not this season. Scrub Arabs.'

Chris went out, not too happy, but a few minutes later was back again, much happier. A small item had come in which was definitely hard stuff. It was rather a mysterious item.

'This wouldn't be Arabs, would it?' Jack said, studying the item.

'Oh, no. She's scrubbed those.'

14

'Compromise on both sides, as part of the piss-making process,' Abo said.

'Abo,' Frank said, cutting in on his headphones. 'Say "peace".'

'Peace,' Abo said.

'Try that part again. From Dr Kissinger.'

'Dr Kissinger said that what was needed was compromise on both sides, as part of the piss-making process.'

'Abo.'

'Hello?' Abo said.

'Say "leave".'

'Leave,' Abo said.

'Say "I leave you in peace".'

'I leave you in peace,' Abo said.

'Now read from Dr Kissinger again.'

'Dr Kissinger said that what was needed,' Abo said, 'was compromise on both sides, as part of the piss-making process.'

'Yes. Okay, Abo,' Frank said, and ranged elsewhere.

Difficult case, Abo.

They were all difficult cases here. He had twelve of them. He was seated at his console, switching in and out of the tape-recorders they were mumbling into around the room.

He looked at his watch. Time – oh, God! – for a spot of grammar.

Four of the twelve, he knew, would fall asleep immediately in grammar. The remainder, with a solitary exception, would nod off before the end. The exception was the Jap. This clever little devil was after more grammar than Frank had. He walked about with a frightening book of it, finding paradoxes with which to tax Frank.

The one defence – of which Frank made full use – lay in the near impossibility of understanding a word that came out of him. Despite his astounding brain his mouth seemed to have been formed along lines not meant for Western speech.

Frank had a quick switch-in to see that all was still well in that quarter. The familiar yowling reassured him, so he threw both master switches, stopping all recorders and speaking to everybody at once.

'Okay, team. Beautiful work. Grammar now.'

They dutifully took off their headsets and assembled nearer him, four of them at once snuggling into comfortable positions; the familiar glaze settling on other eyes. From the clever fellow with the big book the accustomed gleam shone out. Oh, well.

77

Frank rambled on about grammar for half an hour, interrupted by the occasional yowl.

'Prizterrus krekyuze verbin cases substantive yow-oo-yong. Eyung?'

'Yes,' Frank said.

'Or ong inacular ominative owyung ingular niaow?'

'Good point, Miki.' And the right one to stop him at. 'Only sorry there isn't time to go into it. Okay, chaps!' he said loudly, and saw Abo come awake with the rest.

He followed Abo to the Ferrari and got in while Abo detached the two parking notices from the windscreen – he collected upwards of twenty a week at £6 a time – and they boomed grandly off to Sloane Square, and round it to Coryton Place.

They ascended together in the lift, Frank rather anxious. It was early yet, not quite four. But he had an appointment with Steve and Artie at five; and Abo had to be got over first.

Abo had the top floor of a splendid mansion. 'Servant out this afternoon,' he said, as they entered it. 'Whisky?'

'Gin. I feel ginny,' Frank said, smacking his lips.

'You make them, Frank. I feel dirty.'

From Abo this could have had a variety of meanings, but Frank knew he was only going to have a shower. One thing about this son of the sands, he was hygienic to a fault.

Frank poured the drinks, with bitters in his own, and walked about pondering the best way to raise the subject. Abo's residence afforded ample areas for walking in. Interior decorators had been at it for months, knocking down large parts and putting in other parts that Abo wanted. He had a taste for mirrors and panelling; also for enormous picture windows. Frank sipped his gin, still pondering, and had a look out. The fire escape was the principal view from the main window. It snaked five floors down.

He could hear Abo warbling distantly, so he poured himself another, and found the right panel, and the gold cigarette box inside, and lit up one of Abo's specials. Always a fine quality of hashish at the prince's.

While doing it, he prudently checked the main mirror. Only

his own reflection showed in it, but he felt for the panel and opened a half of the mirror and went into the room behind.

The camera was closed up to the mirror but not in operation. He looked through the viewfinder to see what it was closed up on. It was on the huge divan in the room outside. All the room could be seen through the two-way mirror.

Frank came out again and closed the panel and sat in one of the jumbo zebra chairs. The style of everything here was so hideous it amounted to a masterpiece. He knew the fault wasn't the interior decorator's. Abo was obstinate. He knew his own mind, and this was its reflection.

'You lit up,' Abo said, coming in sniffing.

'Relaxer. What's new with that camera?'

'Show you later. Send you out of your mind, oo-wah!' Abo said. He was in a crisp towelling robe, very white against his sallow skin; undeniably sexy, Frank thought. A lively, useful performer, the prince. Fickle, though.

'Abo, what is all this nonsense about the film?' he said, deciding on the direct approach, as Abo lit up and sat.

'What nonsense?'

'Giving them those bills back.'

'Why I pay?'

'You said you would.'

'Why?'

Christ. Ancient failings. Frank remembered his father had had affairs with several Arabs – lowlier ones, from Marrakesh or thereabouts – and had damn near killed a few. Fickle.

'Abo, honestly, what is this kind of money to you? You pay that in parking fines.'

'True.' Abo quietly crowed, amused. 'Forget it, Frank.'

'You'll pay?'

'No.'

'Damn it, Abo, it's my film, too. Why do this to me?'

Abo thought. 'Okay. I see.'

'Aren't you having fun? Smashing boys, some of those actors.'

'Boys so-so. Girls better,' Abo said. 'Surprise, those girls, Frank. Good families. Lady This, Lady That. Surprise.'

'Well, there you are.'

'True, know different things. But only one time.'

'How do you mean?'

'I see one girl one time, then no more. Why?'

'H'm.'

Frank divined the difficulty. Boys were boys and girls were girls, and Abo's experience leaned to the former. What Lady This and Lady That obviously needed was a good talking to.

'You think it might be me?' Abo said, anxiously watching.

'Well, it might be, mightn't it?'

Abo's face darkened.

'I could always ask them,' Frank said.

'Oh, no.'

'Best way to find out, Abo.'

'If I don't like to hear?'

'Why wouldn't you?' Frank asked.

'Oh. Well,' Abo said. He had now grown very gloomy.

He got up and poured another drink.

'I mean, if there is some small thing here or there,' Frank said, 'that should be done some other way, why ever not? Might as well know what's on.'

'You think?' Abo said.

'Definitely. Can't know unless we are told, can we?'

'True,' Abo said, more cheerfully.

Frank came to a strict decision on these girls. Jeopardizing the film for such peccadilloes. 'And since we're all in the film together, Abo,' he said, pressing on rather, 'it's foolish not to know everyone thoroughly. It's such a good film, anyway.'

'Is it?' Abo said. 'I don't understand this film, Frank. What story is it?'

'Well,' Frank said, bracing himself for, and then rejecting, the idea of explaining the film to Abo. 'It's about murders.'

'Make plenty money?' Abo was now quite jovial.

'Well, it might. A few weeks ago I'd have said no. Though absolutely the thing for you,' he added hurriedly. 'Princely job, Abo, helping the arts. But with these murders, and the way the newspapers are going on, it could easily make a lot.'

'Million pounds?' Abo said.

'Oh, I don't know about that.'

'Two million?' Abo said, chuckling. He got up and refilled both glasses. 'Come through now, Frank. Show you something.'

He opened the panel, switching on the small light inside, and they went behind the mirror.

The video room was well equipped. Apart from the TV camera, there was the video recorder, the screen, a couple of TV sets, and the control gear. The place was comfortably furnished; a sofa, armchairs, a small bar. The air conditioning quietly hummed.

Abo went to a tape library and selected a couple of spools. He put one on the recorder, and dimmed the light as he sat.

Lady This appeared almost instantly on the screen, examining her features in the mirror. She was out of focus, though recognizable enough, and recognizably not wearing anything. She seemed suddenly to totter vertically upwards, and Abo appeared, grinning. Peals of laughter and imprecations filled the room in quadrophonic sound as her legs straddled Abo's neck. 'Abo, you beast! Put me down. I'll fall!'

Abo turned, on the screen, and paused a while to give the mirror a view of more of Lady This, and jigged a little round the room with her. Abo, too, was as Allah had made him. Then they collapsed on the divan in sharp focus, and some interesting stuff took place, till an altercation ensued, and Abo switched his remote control off. 'Not interesting now,' he said. 'I show you another. Oo-wah, steam up, this one.'

This one was a mixed doubles, and certainly was steamy. He heard Abo by his side begin to giggle slightly in a way that usually presaged a certain something. Frank had no objection. As the complex foursome urged each other on from the loud-speakers all around, he'd steamed up himself.

They had another drink later, and Frank tried again about the film, without getting anything spectacular or immediate out of Abo.

The best that Abo could come up with was, 'I see, Frank. I think, eh?'

Not a lot to tell the chaps, Frank thought.

He bussed down the King's Road, wondering what might be the best thing all round.

What with one thing and another, he knew for certain what was best for the film.

He jumped off the bus at Manresa Road and hurried round the corner to the art school, already a bit late. Steve and Artie were waiting outside. They'd arranged to go to the bar of the Students' Union, opposite: the art school shared it with the university's chemistry department, whose members were usually there in larger numbers. He could see various white-clad chemical figures now, messing about with test tubes through the lighted windows of the laboratories.

Steve and Artie seemed rather silent. He couldn't tell if he'd interrupted a planning session or an argument. However, he took them inside and told them the latest news, and while they mulled it over went and bought the beer.

'Three pints, Honey,' he said to the lady at the bar.

There was still an unpleasant silence when he returned.

'Well, damn it, look,' he said. 'It isn't the end of the world. Two hundred pounds is no fortune.'

'Not if you've got it,' Steve agreed.

'They'll surely let us *look* at the stuff.'

'That's exactly what they won't fugging do,' Artie said.

The results of the night shooting had still not been seen. The discussion went drearily on till Frank came up with his next idea.

'How about Artie trying to rustle up a commercial backer,' he said, 'to look at what we've got?'

'Screw that, too!' Artie said.

'Oh.' Frank realized the source of the silence. 'I only thought, with all these murders –'

'What Artie thinks there,' Steve said, 'is that we probably haven't got enough to –'

'What is this "probably" shit?' Artie asked. 'Am I the only one *into* this film? We're shooting out of sequence. We still have no special effects. The stuff those shit-heads are hanging on to is so vital for any kind of – Oh, Christ!'

'All right, only an idea,' Frank said. 'All we need really is two hundred quid for the time being.'

'That's all,' Artie said.

'Anybody thought of Denny?'

'Denny?' Artie looked at him. 'What about Denny?'

'Hasn't that wily oriental got black money tucked away ready to go to the cleaners . . . Maybe a loan, or an investment?'

'Well, how about that?' Artie said to Steve.

Steve had a drink. 'He wouldn't lend it,' he said.

'Why wouldn't he?'

'How would you guarantee he got it back?'

'An investment, then.'

'Denny invests in stuff he knows about. Jeans.'

'That's all?' Artie said, and let a small silence develop.

On his quarterly trips to Hong Kong and other parts, Denny handled stuff other than jeans. The money resulting from this stuff was the kind that needed cleaning up. It wasn't money that actually went into a bank anywhere.

They thought about this. Blue Stuff was Denny's one retail outlet – a prestigious Chelsea one, to keep him in touch with the fashion end of the trade – but his basic business was that of importer and wholesaler. His warehouse was at Wembley, where Denny also lived. A Chinese partner ran the warehouse.

Steve was so sure it was a non-starter, he couldn't even bother arguing.

But he thought it funny that Frank should have pushed the idea so hard; and that Artie should have gone along with it.

They both knew Denny.

15

'I TELL you, never be manufactuler. All the time headache,' Denny said. He was tapping his own neat head. He applied himself to the tape measure again. 'Twenty-seven, twenty-seven-half, twenty-eight. Ah? See yourself.'

Steve had a try, and then Stanley and Wendy. The flare of the jeans worked out variously between twenty-seven and twenty-eight inches.

'Dow!' Denny said. He kicked out with his right foot, the only suggestion so far that he was delighted and not in a towering rage. Never easy to tell with Denny.

'That van is hooting a lot out there,' Wendy said.

Not only the van; several cars, unwisely stuck behind it, were also hooting. The King's Road was busy at eleven in the morning.

'Won't hoot long. All back!' Denny said.

'What – aren't we trying the rest?' Stanley said.

'All back. What they think – Oxford Stleet?' Denny said. 'King's Load here. Extleme fashion. All back. Shit!'

The three assistants repacked the few samples measured and put them back in the cartons. Steve and Stanley had carried in six of the cartons, weighing damn near a hundred pounds apiece. They carried them back out again, and after an altercation with the van-man returned to find Denny impassively kicking out with his foot again.

It had certainly put him in a good mood, Steve saw, and he cheered up. Denny did this from time to time, trying out the cheaper English manufacturers against his own imports. If the stuff came up to specification he took it in good part, even though it cost him more.

There was a reckless gambler's quality to him that was quite engaging. He moved with a little lurching walk like some buccaneer of the China Seas. His egg-smooth face with its tiny nose puckered occasionally, but whether with uncontrollable anger or sudden hilarity it was impossible to say. The foot was the thing to watch for, or the sudden fist bunched in the air.

He was going about now saying 'Dow!'

'Denny,' Steve said, 'I wonder if I could have a chat with you today.' It was Friday, when Steve worked all day.

'Not more lise? Had lise.'

'Not a rise, Denny. Business matter, actually.'

'Business, fine. You want to come in full time, Steve?'

'Well, actually what I wanted –'

'Good boy, Steve. I watch you. Make small joke. Good salesman always make small joke. You want that, Steve?'

'Certainly like to think about it, Denny,' Steve said, removing a denim cap from his head. Denny had a funny way of trying out his stock on the staff as he spoke. 'But what I wanted to discuss at the moment –'

'Crever boy. Come here one moment.' Denny was nodding him into a corner. 'How you rike I make manager? I see how customers rike you. Stanley no good, no joke. You work hard, make prenty money, ah?'

Steve removed another cap from his head, and thought. If the promotion could be cemented with a loan, how long would he have to hang on to the job, anyway?

'Won't talk now. Talk rater. Upstairs,' Denny said.

Stanley was walking suspiciously over.

'You want that stuff brought down, then, Denny?' he said.

Stanley had protuberant eyes, which missed little; also a big Adam's apple and an adenoidal voice, none of which Denny liked.

'Okay, I come show you,' Denny said, impassive face registering neither like nor dislike.

A consignment of their own stuff had arrived not many days before. It was still packed in the big bales, and they got it down from the upper shelves with the small block and tackle. There was no need to measure any of this stuff, but Denny did measure a bit, for sheer pleasure. Every one went thirty inches. 'Extleme,' he said.

The early luncheers began drifting in at twelve-thirty. Denny remained in high spirits.

'Little bastard's in his rutting season,' Stanley said, as they watched him take money from a blonde. When in London, Denny alone took money in the shop. When not, his Chinese partner Chen came and took it. 'He'll be doing a few in-seams today, you watch.'

'Stanley, you're awful,' Wendy said, passing at that moment.

Stanley was awful, but right enough here, Steve saw. In cheerful mood, the chairman did show increased activity on the inseam front. The term was a trade one for inside leg measurement, and Denny did it in the largest, lockable, fitting room below. He preferred willowy blondes, and showed uncanny perception for those not averse to in-seam research.

'Ay-ay,' Stanley said presently, as the chairman lurched impassively below, arms full of jeans, in the wake of a likely number. Stanley's Adam's apple was oscillating, his protuberant eyes hungry. He'd never quite mustered the nerve to try himself.

Stanley had some other theories, to do with black dollars, about the large fitting room, probably also correct; certainly Denny was always closeted there with his partner after returns from the orient.

Steve objected to none of this and only rejoiced to see the chairman so cheerful. His opportunity came in the dead period after three.

'Come upstairs now, Steve,' Denny said.

Denny's office was behind the stock room. To make room for extra shelving, the ceiling had been removed, all the rafters visible in Denny's room, too. The place was quite cheerful. Long banners with flights of duck, and calligraphy, gracefully twirled.

Denny seated himself behind his desk.

'Sit, Steve. Been thinking a rot.'

Steve sat. The chairman's face was puckered.

'People in this country razy. Need somebody English with *energy*, blain. Might make partner. In China people work hard. Might take you there, show you. Make there, sell here. Big scale. Biggest. Whatever you want to do. Ah?'

'Well, Denny, that's very handsome, but –'

'I know. You want films. Understand. Young man, actlesses. Understand. But needs *business*, Steve. Needs money. Fantastic business here – only beginning. Whatever you want – chain stores? Make chain. Crever young man. With me together – dow !'

'Well, damn it, Denny, I don't know what to say . . .'

'Come here, Steve. Just rook down there.'

He had stood and gone to the window, and Steve joined him.

The King's Road slowly swarmed below in autumnal sunlight.

'Brue, ah?'

'Brue?'

'Every one. Brue stuff. No Chairman Mao here. Do it all themselves. Ah?'

He turned and resumed his seat, and so did Steve.

Denny now stared very impassively, saying nothing.

Steve realized that the crunch had come, and panted a little.

'What is actually bugging me at the moment,' he said, 'is that I'm stuck in this film and we need two hundred pounds.'

Denny maintained the silence.

'Which isn't very much,' Steve said. He looked frantically all over Denny's face in search of some expression. Not a trace showed. 'That's what's bugging me,' he said.

'Disappointed, Steve,' Denny said at last.

'Well, it's a proposition, Denny. Over a year's work, you know. Night and day. Have to finish with it.'

Denny got up and went to the window, and came back and sat down again. 'What ploposition?' he said.

'I wondered, firstly, if you'd lend it.'

'Not a money-render,' Denny said.

'Alternatively, invest it.'

'Don't invest what I don't know.'

'Only two hundred quid. Say four hundred dollars. In notes,' Steve said, pushing it a bit. 'Not much, is it, Denny?'

Denny stared longer.

'What dollars?' he said.

'Four hundred.'

'Why dollars?'

'Two hundred quid.'

After a pause, Denny said, 'Disappointed, Steve.'

'Denny, you said you understood. If you understand that I'm stuck in this thing –'

'Understand,' Denny said.

Nothing much had happened to his face, but some damned thing had happened. It had switched off.

Steve put in a last effort.

He said, 'Look, Denny, I don't understand business. But you weren't looking for a business brain, were you?'

'No. I business blain,' Denny said.

'It *needs* your sort of brain. Let Artie come and explain the facts and figures to you. He's got all that stuff. I mean, there *is* money in it, I'm sure. And we've done so much.'

Denny opened a drawer and took out a diary.

'Wednesday,' he said.

'It's only Friday now, Denny.'

'Seven o'crock. No, Chen is coming. Seven-thirty. Wednesday.'

Denny didn't say any more, and he didn't seem to expect Steve to say any more.

They returned silently to the shop together.

They worked late Friday and Steve felt distinctly knackered as he left. He'd brooded all afternoon over his handling of the interview, and he knew he shouldn't have mentioned dollars. Still, his expectations hadn't been high.

He bought a *Globe* in the street.

SCOTLAND YARD BAFFLED ran the headline, and above it two other racing lines: *Is mad genius behind Chelsea killings? As coded notes reach police ...*

Still standing in the street, he read the first bold paragraph.

A deranged genius may be responsible for the recent spate of murders in Chelsea. News exclusive to the Evening Globe *indicates that the police have received 'coded notes' revealing detailed knowledge of the pattern of murder. Although Scotland Yard would neither confirm nor deny the report, evidence of an 'extraordinary intelligence' is believed to be shown by ...*

Steve read on, all down the column, fascinated.

Frank read it, too, similarly fascinated.

So did Artie.

And Mooney.

As was soon obvious, the C.C. had read it, too.

'Well, Ted,' he said on the phone. 'Where did they get it?'

'Inquiries going on now.'

'Information Room here is a madhouse at the moment. We need a discussion, Ted.'

88

'Ng,' Warton said.

'Can't have you here. They'll think you're being carpeted. Are you getting the Press there any more?'

'A few hanging about at the moment. Waiting for me to leave, I expect.'

'Do you expect 'em in the morning?'

'*Tomorrow* morning?'

'I'm prepared to give up a Saturday. Are you?'

'Well, naturally, sir,' Warton said slowly.

'Let's leave it till noon. They'll have gone by then. I'll drive myself, private car.'

'Fine, sir. And thank you.'

Warton hung up and considered. Coming to Chelsea. Could easily have seen him at some neutral location. Wanted to see the procedure, Incident Room. That was perfectly okay. Wouldn't find a better one anywhere.

He was uneasy, though.

What he had expected to happen hadn't happened yet.

16

DESPITE his strong dislike for the job, Warton was a considerable innovator in it. He had to go about and see bodies, which was offensive enough, but apart from this, he believed in placing himself at several removes from the actuality of crime; of sanitizing himself. This called for a pretty strong sanitation squad, and one of the hallmarks of a Warton investigation was both the size of his field force and of the administrative staff to back it up.

Like Montgomery of El Alamein, he believed in numbers; and the proper use of them meant efficient communications and a well-run Incident Room. He hadn't himself invented the latter term, but he'd invented many of the procedures now standard in criminal investigation departments everywhere.

Few carried them out as formidably as Warton himself.

On out-of-town jobs, his first demand was for the installation of twenty extra phones; then for the drafting in of staff to man them, and secretaries to type the information, and clerks to index it.

In the metropolitan area this wasn't often necessary; and at Chelsea the headquarters were almost to his own design. All he'd had to do was send Summers along to open the suite of rooms, take the locks off the phones, and start the Journal.

All the rest, on his standing instructions (pasted into the front of the Journal), automatically followed: the checking of the Telex link with Scotland Yard's computer, the delivery of office machines and stationery, arrangements for twenty-four-hour canteen facilities, and so on.

A case sergeant, under Summers's direct instructions, was the second draftee; and the investigation was under way. It was the function of the case sergeant to keep the Cumulatives. There were two of them, one a simple narrative, summarized from the Journal, and the second the annotated one which detailed Main Card numbers for the cross-filing index.

The filing system, a reflection of Warton's very soul, broke things down exceeding small. There were cards for everything.

There was a card for *Pickles* (as missing from Miss Jane Manningham-Worsley's).

There was a card for *Semen* (as removed from Miss J.M.W.).

There was a card for *Spit*. A spit-test had been carried out on the husband and also the eldest son of Miss J.M.W.'s daily; saliva an accurate guide to semen.

There was a series of cards for Miss J.M.W.'s bank-drawings over a period of three years. The daily had said that no sums were missing; but had the old lady drawn sums which she had not used?

From the cards it was possible to see, to within about fifteen minutes, what every resident of Bywater Street had been doing on the night when Alvin C. Schuster had been wrapped round the lamp-post.

Warton didn't believe much in flair or hunch; all the same it was his way to sit and try to visualize the circumstances of a crime. In the case of A. C. Schuster he had visualized a jolly-ole-pal threesome proceeding along Bywater Street, deceased

Schuster as middle man. (Card, *Drunks*.) Or a car reversing rapidly down one-way Bywater Street for the minute or two necessary to deposit Schuster; with another car blocking the entrance so that exit was guaranteed. (Cards, *Reversing Vehicles; Obstructing Vehicles; Taxis – Reports*.)

Even in the case of a lady so limited socially as Miss J.M.W. there were upwards of 150 cards. Schuster ran to over 700; Germaine to over 1800. This was because of her gregarious nature, and the Colbert-Greer connection; and through him, the film operation with its many ramifications.

Colbert-Greer's movements, within a period of one hour and ten minutes, had alone filled twenty-seven cards, including one detailing the radio programme that Mrs Hester Bulstrode had been listening to when rudely interrupted in the lavatory. Mrs B. had half a dozen cards to herself; her landlord, Mr Shankar B. Singh, had three. The central heating firm replacing the defective boiler on the premises had two cards. The old lady had complained of the boiler to Singh (one of his cards), and also, of the inflammation risk, to the Borough Surveyor and Goshawk Road police station (two further cards).

The cards revealed everything; and they also revealed Warton, and the reason why this dogged man would not easily be deflected from what he wanted.

What he wanted was a nice room at New Scotland Yard supervising some general aspect of Order; with respectability, and regularity, and anonymity, and a vase of flowers from his garden. And he bloody meant to get it.

So he was up in good time next day, giving himself a careful shave, and a steady look. His hand was pretty steady, too, though he was nervous.

He deliberately didn't ring Lucan Place, and he took his time getting there. But he still managed it by eleven-thirty.

What he had expected to happen had still not happened.

*

The C.C. was the soul of affability in the Incident Room. He was in a tweed jacket and slacks. So was Warton, and so was Summers. Several of the young shits were in jeans, of course;

still, matter of form these days, and they were all plain-clothes men, and it was Saturday after all.

'Very interesting. Lot on this fellow Artie Johnston.'

'The blackie, sir. Mentioned him.'

'*Rocking with Rimbaud*, eh?'

'Book of poetry he wrote.'

'M'm.'

'Other one interested in poetry, too, sir,' Summers volunteered. 'Colbert-Greer.'

'So I see.'

'The poetry of a particular *period*, sir. It's known as the Pre-Raphaelite period,' Summers solemnly offered.

'Yes. I've heard of it.'

'Involving *Rossetti*.'

'Quite.'

Warton silently seethed. What Summers needed was his arse kicking; preening like this; Saturday or no Saturday.

'Why all the cross-references to "Shaft"?' the C.C. said.

Warton waited one moment, silently glowering, to see if Summers felt like pirouetting up and down the room while explaining this one; but he evidently read the look and said nothing.

'It's a gay club, sir, both sexes,' Warton said. 'Germaine Roberts was a member. So is Colbert-Greer. We've got a few things going forward there. Adjacent to Cremorne Wharf.'

'Ah.'

The C.C. dutifully examined the waiting murder bags, and the Journal, continuously being compiled from the chits that were handed in, and said, 'Well, Ted.'

'Yes, sir.'

'Care for coffee, sir?' was Summers's final fling.

'Why not? Thanks.'

'Ng,' Warton said. Rough time for Summers next week.

The two of them went through to Warton's room, where as a matter of course, and quite casually, the C.C. took the superintendent's chair behind the desk, and Warton seated himself in the visitor's chair.

'Now then, Ted,' said the C.C. 'Perhaps you'd favour me with your views.'

Both the tone and the content of this remark lowered Warton's spirits, which had been sinking at a rapid rate anyway.

What he had expected hadn't happened. He had confidently counted on – would have pledged his pension on – the arrival of another quotation. Clever bastards like this didn't stop. They couldn't, any more than boozers or drug addicts. Forty-eight hours was the average time Warton would have given him, seventy-two the maximum. He'd hung around last night waiting for the next quotation.

Well, where was it?

He'd been so sure, he'd taken the trouble to indent for an *Oxford Dictionary of Quotations*, and to browse through for the expected shafts of wit. Miss J.M.W. would evidently produce a few pithy words from J. M. Whistler; A. C. Schuster a fiery dart from Algernon C. Swinburne.

But nothing had come.

'Well, sir,' he said heavily, 'we established – fairly rapidly, I may say – that all three people the girl in the library told could have seen the list the following day. Colbert-Greer, of course, worked in the same room –'

'Quite. This newspaper report, Ted.'

'Well, my view there, sir . . .' Warton said. 'You'll recall it was the *Globe* that sprang the story.'

'Yes, I can recall that.'

'Almost certainly supplied by their stringer on the *Chelsea Gazette*. A girl called Mooney. Now, she's been pretty solidly covering this film, which seems to imply that all three were quite well –'

'You're not suggesting the chap is *telling* her what he's doing?'

'No, sir, no,' Warton said, sweating, and at that moment was interrupted by bloody Summers with the coffee.

Except it wasn't coffee.

Summers, looking like one o'clock struck, had some familiar stuff in his hands; a white envelope and a sheet of cartridge paper. Barely listening to the babbling coming out of him,

Warton took it, between the two pieces of Kleenex with which
it was proffered. Four lines of Letraset Gothic:

> Stolen sweets
>   are always sweeter,
> Stolen kisses
>   much completer.

Well, thank you, God, Warton thought devoutly.

'Just arrived?' he said pleasantly.

'Yes, sir. Posted last night. Some mess-up at the post office
that we can't quite –'

'Coffee coming?'

'Yes, sir. But I thought –'

'Whenever it's ready,' Warton said, snout indicating the doorway through which, with all expedition, Summers might now
take himself off; which he did, still silently chiming thirteen.

The C.C. seemed to be chiming, too.

'No fingers if you *don't* mind, sir,' Warton said, offering it.

He was already reaching for the *Oxford*.

'What is it?' the C.C. said.

'Another from our friend, I rather fancy,' Warton said. And
top o' the morning to *you*, sir, he silently added.

Kisses, eh?

Old Algernon was the hot one for kisses.

Kiss; Kissed; Kisses . . .

He went down the column.

Stolen k. much completer.   266:1.

He turned adeptly to page 266, quotation 1.

> Stolen sweets are always sweeter,
>   Stolen kisses much completer,
> Stolen looks are nice in chapels,
>   Stolen, stolen, be your apples.
> > 'Song of Fairies Robbing an Orchard'.
> > *Leigh Hunt.*

'Fairies robbing an orchard?' the C.C. said.

'*Leigh Hunt?*' said Warton.

'I'm not sure that I –'

'Can't be. It's got to be Algernon. Or Whistler. It's got to be, hasn't it?'

'Eh?' the C.C. said.

Warton was racing through Kisses again.

> *Stolen k. much completer.*   266:1.

Fairies robbing the bloody orchard, all right! But who was this Hunt? How had he sneaked in? Was he even on the Residents' List? A swift check showed Hunt's credentials in order there.

> *HUNT, Leigh. Essayist & Poet.*
> *22 Upper Cheyne Row, Chelsea.*

But this was crazy. On the Residents' List; not on the Murder List. Not on *their* murder list, anyway. Feeling himself beginning to chime not just thirteen, but fourteen and fifteen, Warton realized that events had taken a slightly new turn.

The advice note here was for a murder not yet delivered.

'Coffee, sir?' Summers said, bloodhounding in.

A few minutes later, Warton was putting a lifetime's concentration into trying to keep his face straight. He was well aware of the gravity of the event, but the manner of it was so delightful, a few moments' enjoyment was surely in order.

In the twinkling of an eye, without need for plea or argument, the contents of his plate had been transferred to the C.C.'s plate. The switch was so dexterous, so supernaturally swift and dire, it might almost have been ordained by some great Incident Room above. Huge pinnacles of crap seemed silently to form and re-form on the C.C.'s plate, fresh accretions joining by the moment. The C.C. didn't, as yet, seem to realize what was happening on his plate.

Well, give him a minute, Warton thought.

'What's your view, Ted?'

'Ng,' Warton said neutrally, sipping his coffee.

'Practical joke?'

'Same joker, if so.'

'What do you intend doing about it?'

'Well,' Warton said, and cleared his throat. Begin count-down. Ten, nine, eight . . . 'Have to take instructions from you on this one, sir.'

'Instructions? What instructions?'

'Question of policy, sir.'

Seven, six, five . . .

'What policy?'

'Press.'

'Would you like to be more specific, Ted?'

Certainly would.

'You'll want to publish, will you, sir?'

'Eh?'

Four, three, two, one . . .

Blast-off! We have a launch. We have a perfect launch. Hoo-hoo-hoo! Top o' the morning.

'Or won't you want to publish, sir?'

'Oh.'

That's it. Got it. Now, I want to see every bit of that crap eaten up. Eat up all your nice crap and you'll grow up into a fine useful little crap-eater.

'Well, in the case of a practical *joke*,' the C.C. said, anxiously scanning Warton's face.

Warton offered nothing at all.

'What would you do, Ted?'

'Feel bound to apply to you for instructions, sir.'

'Well, I'll, uh, turn this over in my mind, Ted.'

That's the form. Also in the bowels. Relaxing week-end re-commended. Somewhere like Tibet. Take the pressure off.

'Much appreciate your coming in, sir.'

'I'll call you, uh, tonight, Ted. Be in, I hope?'

'Oh, yes,' Warton said, face immense with gravity. 'Very serious matter.'

'Yes. Yes,' the C.C. said, and went on quietly murmuring it as he was escorted from the premises. Warton watched the dazed figure entering his car in Lucan Place, and nodded.

Knew that feeling.

17

Mooney altered her voice whenever the *Globe* rang that week-end, which was often, to let them know she wasn't in.

Nothing was going off at half-cock this time. People had to take what was good for them; couldn't have all their chocolate at once.

She'd seen the mileage they'd got out of her item on Friday. The Saturdays showed the field in full cry; and the police had said nothing. She hadn't expected them to. No, all hers at the moment. And a first-class moment.

A nasty one, true, had come from Wertmuller. Her moves on the rapture front had been planned for Sunday, but he rang on Saturday to say he had to go to Huddersfield to see an Atkinson.

'A what?'

'A harp, Mary. A most beautiful specimen. It needs restoring.'

'Oh, does it?' Mooney said, dully.

'It's a great privilege, Mary,' Wertmuller told her seriously, 'just to be asked to lay hands on such an instrument.'

'Well, in that case –'

'Mary, if you wish me to leave the Atkinson –'

'Of course I don't. You *must* go and lay hands on it. I won't hear another word,' Mooney said, knowing pretty well what would happen to the Atkinson if she laid hands on it.

'Can our evening still take place – perhaps on Monday?'

'Of course it can, Otto.'

'Ah. I'll just wait till then, Mary, dear.'

Well, damn it, just listening to him was a benison. And after all it was only two days to – whacko! – Monday. Then the great restorer could really crack on.

Meanwhile, she had plenty to occupy her.

So did Frank, who had an interesting wheeze of his own going just then. He'd made a new chum at Shaft, so it was a busy week-end all round.

And the same for Artie, who continued dishing out the duck, *Chez Georges*, without allowing it to interfere with his other plans.

Steve carried on selling jeans all Saturday, and all Sunday carried on with what was best for Steve.

Abo just carried on having a lovely time.

Warton put in some hours at the office, and then some more in the garden, thinking steadily.

His spirits darkened as he thought.

His correspondent, whoever he was, was either having a game with him, or seriously planning a murder. He couldn't tell which.

The message had to be taken seriously, in any case.

L.H. of Chelsea had to be contacted and warned. A glance through the telephone directory, with its close-packed Halls, Hammonds and Harrisons, and the numbers of them with L initials, had already shown phoning not to be a valid way of doing this; even if everyone in Chelsea was connected to a phone.

An early thought was that the message might portend action at joke level. It might herald an In Memoriam announcement; perhaps for Leigh Hunt himself. The dates had proved unlikely here (Hunt was found to have died in August 1859, and it was now late October); however, the idea had suggested a valid procedure, so Warton had written out a chit.

First thing Monday morning, all classified ads booked in the London dailies and in the local press would be checked. (Cover: fraud or public mischief, at Summers's discretion.)

He had set some other procedures going at joke level.

At fatality level there was only one procedure: publication.

There were such stunning arguments against this, that as he got the wallflowers (now very stalky) out of their boxes and into the ground, Warton simply wished the C.C. the best of luck.

First and foremost was that if no attack took place, it would show the C.C. as a colossal bloody idiot. It would produce not only the alarm he wished to avoid, but a harvest of similar warnings from that brigade who regularly dispatched hearses to people still alive and fire engines to places not on fire.

All would have to be investigated; grossly misusing man-power, muddying trails.

And there were some good trails. Steady work had already identified where paper and lettering might have come from.

The paper, of limited make and discontinued style, had gone four years ago to just two London wholesalers apart from the main art schools.

All the art schools' supplies had been exhausted long ago. The wholesalers had none left, but two art shops in the King's Road, Winsor & Newton's, and Brierley Bros., still had some.

The type style had proved unexpectedly more difficult. Though unusual, small quantities had been widely dispersed, and some hundreds of man-hours had gone into tracking it down. What had been established was that within a fifteen-mile radius, only two outlets had it; Chelsea Art School, and Brierley Bros.

More to the point, Brierley's old-fashioned duplicate invoice book showed that six sheets of cartridge paper and six sheets of Letraset, type unknown, had been sold on Wednesday morning. The dozy assistant whose initials were on the carbon copy couldn't remember the sale, and as stock-keeping was not up to par, there was no other evidence.

Still, Warton's money was on Brierley's.

It was near the post office. It was notably disorganized and dusty. It had both sets of materials and actually a specimen of Letraset Gothic still curling in the window.

Not conclusive, of course, but nothing was conclusive here.

There was an abstract glee about the messages that disturbed him. The sender had a special point to make: a person not bound by normal considerations. A dangerous person.

He thought that par for the course, as far as the C.C. was concerned, would be about ten o'clock. He'd ring by then.

The C.C. rang at a couple of minutes to.

'I think we have to take it as a practical joke, Ted?'

Warton caught the interrogative, but he simply said, 'I see, sir.'

'After the nonsense in the Information Room, it would look as if we're being particularly sensitive – h'm?'

'Ng.'

99

'You don't take it seriously, then?'

'I do. I take it very seriously.'

'Well, that's my view at the moment.'

'Appreciate your telling me, sir,' Warton said, and hung up, pleased at his forecast; at the same time even more disturbed by it.

The young lady with the head had two weeks to go then.

He got in early on Monday, and the Incident Room quite soon began to come up with items.

The classified columns of the *Telegraph* were due to carry a four-liner for a Lancelot Horniman who had taken off after sufferings bravely borne (no flowers); and the *Chelsea News* was to commemorate in its Friday issue the tenth anniversary of the death of Leslie Hoop (We linger here with Thoughts so Sad, As constantly we Mourn you, Dad): both genuine.

The evenings, when they arrived, were a bit of a mystery. *News* and *Standard* both niggly, though naturally sketchy so early in the day: they carried the same agency photo of Mrs Thatcher chatting up a young copper outside her door. The *Globe* was strangely subdued; little piece by their bloke Packer, obviously written after Friday's shenanigans in the Yard's Information Room.

Something must be going on there.

*

'Damn it, tell her I want to speak to her myself.'

'Well, I'll *try*, Jack.'

'What is this bloody uppity nonsense?'

'She can't blow her sources, Jack, is what she's –'

'On the *paper*, she can't blow them?'

'She isn't on the paper. That's what she's –'

'Put her on that bloody phone right away. Isn't there any bloody loyalty in the world? If I make myself bloody clear?'

'Crystal bloody clear, Jack.'

But when Chris got through, Mooney said she couldn't speak just then; which was the case, because not only Len Offard

(*Sun*), but Pip Stewart and Rex Goddard and Sheila Cohen (stringers, respectively, for the *Express*, *News* and *Guardian*) were all watching her like hawks from the double-banked lines of roll-top desks. So she hopped round the corner, and called Jack from a phone box there.

On the two occasions that she'd previously spoken to him, she'd had to wait ten minutes. He was in her ear immediately now.

'*Mary!*' Jack said. 'What are your problems, darling?'

'You see, Jack,' Mooney said huskily, using his given name for the first time, 'it's very difficult for –'

'You have to understand how we're fixed, Mary. With a story like this, one has absolutely got to piss or get off the pot. We *must* have more, darling. Now, I want you to come in and see me right away.'

'Well, if it's humanly –'

'Have you got more?'

'I'm getting it. I can't –'

'From police sources?'

'No. Really, Jack, I –'

'*Maniac* sources?'

Mooney had a quick double-take. Maniac?

'It's so delicate, Jack,' she said, almost instantaneously, 'that I'd sooner you didn't press. I don't feel free to –'

'Feel free,' Jack said. 'I want you to. If there's any *professional* problem, I want it sorted out. We can't get stuck like this! I hope you're getting the point, Mary. If there's something you particularly want, you have my assurance –'

Mooney got the point, but she wanted better assurances, and at another time, so she said urgently, 'I'm going now.'

'*Mary!*' Jack hollered. 'You're sure of those notes?'

'Absolutely.'

'There hasn't been another, has there?'

'Yes,' Mooney said, after the slightest pause. 'But –'

'Oh, my God, bloody come *in* here, darling! . . . Darling?'

But Mooney had hung up, and was looking through the dusty glass into humdrum Fulham, with a feeling of distinct unease.

She hadn't meant to mention other notes.

However, she had, and at the *Globe* a new front page took shape.

Warton heard about it a couple of hours before he saw it.

The C.C. didn't call himself. He put Warton's immediate superior, a Commander, on to the job.

'Their chap Packer here has been asking questions, Ted. Where are they getting it from?'

'A girl called Mooney, their stringer. I told the C.C.'

'Where is she getting it?'

'Give me a direct order, sir, and I'll ask her. That would mean confirming her stuff. Which is why I want the direct order.'

'Okay, I'll see what I can do.'

But no order came, so Warton did nothing; and in the afternoon the *Globe* did.

MANIAC: HE SIGNALS AGAIN.

Warton read thoroughly through the stuff. All innuendo and barrel scrapings. They hadn't got much, but they'd evidently got something. He wondered at the primary source of even this little.

He stayed till a quarter-to seven, and went home, and had just entered the house when the phone rang for him.

Rose had barely taken his mac, and she stood with it watching as, with a strange half-scowl which she knew to be a sign of satisfaction, he said, 'That so? Is that a first name or – Ng. Mrs, eh? Okay. Coming in.'

Mrs Louisa Honey was the latest. Manresa Road, Chelsea.

18

HONEY was a cleaner in the chemistry labs of Chelsea College, but she also put in a couple of evenings at the bar of the Students' Union. There was a social that night (a birthday), but she had only been able to stay till seven.

As she hurried out in the dark, an arm came round her waist.

Some of the students had been a bit high when she'd left. She said, 'Here – cheeky young devil!' and turned.

As she did so, another hand covered her face.

She gazed up, astonished. A huge head loomed above her. It had an open cupid's mouth, radiantly smiling; and rank upon rank of finely waved hair.

As she drew breath to scream, she felt her senses going. Just before she passed out, the cupid's mouth bent tenderly to her own.

She was still hysterical when Warton saw her, in her flat at World's End at half-past eight.

'Chloroformed, sir,' the sergeant said.

The police doctor had already seen her; she was mildly sedated but still coming out with small whooping cries.

It had been someone 'ever so tall'. He had had a big hair style and a face of peculiar chalky whiteness (mask?).

With the odd 'ng' here and there, Warton had built up a fairly complete picture.

The person who was ever so tall was also very slim; there was a funny smell about him, hardly like a man at all. Warton had asked if she'd ever had chloroform before, and apparently she hadn't. While she was swooning away, this tall person had continued kissing her. His lips were horrible, like rubber. In view of Honey's distinctly homely appearance, some eyebrows were raised at this.

Warton's conclusion was that her account was accurate. He thought that the tall person with the chalky white face and the rubbery lips had certainly given her a kiss, and also an insufficient whiff of chloroform on a pad.

He pushed his way through the Pressmen in the courtyard of the tenement block, and later found another gang of them at his HQ. When he emerged, it was almost eleven, and the reporters were still waiting for him. Many local stringers had been alerted and were also present; but their ranks did not include Mooney.

Mooney, by then, was into a different scene.

*

Wertmuller had arrived prompt at eight with a bunch of chrysanthemums.

He seemed more massive than ever in the small flat, and also rather awkward and constrained. A glass of sherry didn't do much to improve this, so Mooney put a slug of Martell into him, and also in to herself.

This seemed the right fuel, and after another (with a graceful exit to keep the oven under control), she had him humming along; harps and Huddersfield, harmony and Hamburg.

She'd hesitated over what background music to put on. The classics seemed to be coming it a bit, even Vivaldi, which she'd ringed him as, but something along gentle ballad lines couldn't hurt; so a clutch of troubadours discreetly alighted one after the other on to the turntable.

As they inoffensively warbled, and fantastic Otto, as she noticed, got mildly pissed, she stationed herself companionably nearer him, though at a lower level, in fact on the floor, where without inconvenience he could knead a little if the inclination took him, and she could rest her glass on his knee. In no time at all one long finger was stroking her wrist, and a whole handful of them her hair.

All this was so exactly what was ordered, by way at least of a relish, that she could fairly hear herself purring. He talked about his work, and the German scene, and how, professionally, the English was incomparably better; he confided he was really here to take lessons.

'Are you, Otto? You didn't mention that.'

'The shop asked me not to, Mary. I didn't want to keep it from you. They thought it would be bad for business,' he said, twinkling, 'if you wrote that I was simply a student.'

'But you're more than that.'

Well, he was; but for these specialized restorations, the work rooms of the Victoria & Albert Museum were where one had to go and learn. 'You won't write it?' he said.

'Of course I won't.' But at mention of the magic names, a pang had gone through her. She'd been groping for just the image; something romantically German, well pre-jackboot, mildly tutorial, in general terms gorgeous. Albert. Her Prince

Albert. And Otto was a better name than Albert, and Mrs Otto better still. Mrs Otto W. Well, damn it, Mooney thought, and had a job keeping her hands out of his hair.

To give them something to do, and since the stuff was doing such a great job, she uncoiled herself upwards and poured out another couple of slugs.

He had a further surprise for her when she turned. From a breast pocket he had removed something like a paper-wrapped bread stick.

'For you,' he said, shyly proffering it, 'if you like it.'

'For me?'

'If you truly like it, Mary.'

Wonderingly, she unwound the wrapping to reveal, somewhat mystifyingly, a rather dicey little flute, much battered.

'Oh, well, my goodness,' she said, working hard at liking it, 'it's lovely.'

'I will make it so. It's a *Löwenherz*, Mary.'

'*Is it?*' Mooney said, almost falling over.

'Oh, there is no doubt – a genuine Löwenherz. Only think, little Lotte found it for me at a bazaar, she is so clever.'

She had been hearing of this Lotte, the only blot on the horizon so far; his small musical sister who seemed a bloody sight too clever for her years.

'In a Löwenherz we find great purity of tone,' Otto instructed.

'Do we?' Mooney said. God, he was marvellous.

'If you could – have we some other music?'

Had she! She practically destroyed Leonard Cohen and Bob Dylan in her haste to get Vivaldi at it.

'Ah. Very good,' he said. 'The gigue.'

He held the thing horizontally and blew, and did indeed get some very nice tones. He smiled and nodded as he did this, and she smiled and nodded along, until excessive nodding from his direction indicated that she was intended to dance along rather than simply nod along.

Ever willing, she hitched up her skirt an inch and prettily obliged, until it occurred to her that six-footers didn't show to tremendous advantage doing a jig in a small room, so after a second or two more of thudding about, she packed it in. 'I don't know what I'm thinking of,' she explained. 'You must be ravenous. We can jig a bit later.'

This could have been better expressed, it occurred to her, en route to the kitchen, but the nuance had escaped him, and he was looking professionally enough at the Löwenherz as she returned.

She fed him his shrimp cocktail, and he exclaimed properly enough over her chicken casserole; very good, though she said it herself. It was his turn to let her know what was what in the matter of the Hock, and hers to instruct him on syllabubs.

He was rather a glutton for interesting facts, as she was herself, and they had rather a feast of them in the candle-light. In this light she knew she was looking by no means bad, and he himself so absolutely whacko that for lengthy periods she didn't attend to what his delicious voice was actually saying.

They'd been going there and back over the relative advantages of life in Germany and England. For herself, Mooney didn't care if they lived in the forest, like Hansel and Gretel; or in Timbuctu, come to that. But it apparently depended upon instructional and professional facilities.

'Ah, Mary, it is so good to talk to you,' he said, stroking her hand. 'To have somebody I *can* talk to.'

'Is it, Otto?'

'Wonderful. Always, always I have wanted a sister.'

'Well, you've got one, haven't you?'

'Ah, Lotte. My *little* sister.' With a rather secretive smile he was taking a photo out of his wallet. 'But always I wanted an older sister. You are her, Mary.'

She'd had sherry and brandy and wine, but it couldn't be that, could it? In some bemusement, Mooney looked at the photo he was showing. A photo of her?

It wasn't of her.

'Who's this?' she said.

'Elke. My fiancée. Isn't she beautiful?'

The little blonde cow was smirking away in the photo.

Mooney didn't know what to do. She didn't know whether to throw it back at him, or tear it up, or simply to tip up the whole table in his lap.

His stupid slow voice was belling out the awful phrases.

'We will be married, but what, for her musical education, is the best? Here undoubtedly ... her mother ... my father ... the professional possibilities ... all my life someone to whom I can really talk ... Ah, Mary, dear, don't you love her?'

'I'm tired,' Mooney said.

'Ah!' He was immediately attentive. 'You have worked today.'

'That's right.' Like a dog. And other days, getting the ingredients for his sodding casserole.

He was enormously contrite. 'I will go now.'

She didn't stop him. She didn't wrestle him to the floor, or kick him in the crutch.

'I will restore the Löwenherz. I knew you'd love it, but after all, we'd talked so little, Mary. It was a question of immediate sympathy. Right away I saw in you that sister – but one has to be certain. I will attach, I think, a little cord, a leather – thang?'

'Thong,' Mooney said.

'Yes. It will go – just so. On this wall, I think. Don't you think that is the best?'

'Yes,' Mooney said.

'Yes. You are tired, Mary dear. I can see it.'

That's right. Like everybody's very oldest sister.

She let him go. She laughed. She cried. She remembered the jig she had danced for him, metaphorically as well as literally. Hansel and Gretel. Mrs O.W. Oh, well. Systematically, she broke the Vivaldi record, and then broke the halves, too. Then she stuffed the chrysanthemums in the bin. As for the flute, he knew where he could stuff that. But still her energy was not spent, and she thought what else to do.

19

THE front pages were black with chloroform next morning. As Jack had said, there was nothing to touch a maniac for keeping readers up to the mark. Like the Boston Strangler and the Cambridge Rapist before him, the Chelsea Maniac now entered the Press pantheon.

He sprang in fully-costumed with his big head and his white face and his rubbery lips; and also with an interesting new set of characteristics. The *Globe* had already established that he was not only a deranged genius but one who mocked the police with coded notes. As every one of the papers noted, the police were still refusing comment, apparently preferring protection of their reputation to that of the public.

Warton, grimly reading, saw that they had a point.

But he brooded on another.

What his correspondent had advised was an intention to steal a kiss; from L.H. What he had demonstrated was that if he had wanted, he could have stolen a life as well; that he had to be taken seriously.

But seriously in which way? What did he want? If it were simply publicity he could have sent the messages to the Press himself. Evidently he didn't wish to do this. But the Press (at least the *Globe*) had in some way got wind of them.

Warton had an itch to call the girl Mooney to find out how; and waited restlessly for the order instructing him to. It hadn't come by mid-day, and he read through the early editions of the evenings, all still heavy with the manic kisser.

A few minutes before one he called the Yard himself, to learn that the C.C. and all senior officers were conferring on the matter; and put down the phone, burning. As the man in charge of the case, shouldn't he be conferring with them?

He had sandwiches in his office, and at two was favoured with a call from his Commander.

'Pull Mooney in, Ted.'

'Right.'

'Have you got up the C.C.'s nose in some way?'

'Wouldn't know,' Warton said.

'Try and be flexible, old boy.'

'Like me to come off the case?' Warton said stiffly.

'Don't be so damn silly. There's nobody better. There are a lot of issues here, Ted. We were discussing them.'

'Yes. Heard you were conferring,' Warton said.

'He knew you were up to the neck. His opening remark – you weren't to be disturbed.'

'I see,' Warton said, somewhat mollified. 'You realize that pulling her in confirms the notes?'

'Go ahead.'

'Okay.' He buzzed Summers and told him to get Mooney.

However, it was Tuesday, and Mooney wasn't so easily to be got; the last pages were due down and she was phoning in stories from here and there.

'Righto. Whenever you do contact her,' Warton said, when Summers came in to explain the delay. 'I'll be waiting.'

He had looked up from the latest editions, with a certain relish. 'Seen the *Globe*, Summers?'

'Yes, sir.'

Too late for its rivals to compete, the *Globe* had suddenly dropped Honey as its main attraction, and had very dramatically and startlingly re-made the paper, widening the field and giving it quite a new and urgent quality.

THE SIEGE OF CHELSEA.

'Not bad,' Warton said. 'Buy it myself. Who's this bloke?' He was tapping the photo of the policeman decorating the page.

'That,' Summers said loweringly, 'is the young prick who was on the door at The Gold Key when the girl removed the photo. I've just been talking to his local station. The *Globe* apparently told them last week they were doing a series on London police, and they fell for it. This – this bloke volunteered.'

Warton gave a low chuckle. He'd thought it too good a production to have been dreamed up in the course of the day; backed up to the hilt inside, special stories: gyms, locksmiths, sex clubs. 'Got on to Shaft, I see.'

'Yes, sir.'

'Got to hand it to them. They do a job. Let me know, then.'

'Yes, sir,' Summers said, and went out; and within the minute was back again.

Warton looked silently at his stricken face, and at what was in his hand.

Then they both looked at it, on his desk.

This one had been posted in a street pillar box some time between mid-day and 3 p.m. when the box had last been emptied.

Same paper, same type style.

> To dance to flutes,
>   To dance to lutes,
> Is delicate
>   And rare.

With the briefest look at Summers, Warton reached for the *Oxford*, and traced the quote.

> It is sweet to dance to violins
>   When love and life are fair;
> To dance to flutes, to dance to lutes
>   Is delicate and rare:
> But it is not neat with nimble feet
>   To dance upon the air!
>   *'The Ballad of Reading Gaol'.*
>   *Oscar Wilde.*

*

All morning, after seeing the papers, Brenda had been feeling nervous, but it wasn't till mid-afternoon that she braced herself.

'Could I have a word with you?' she asked the chief librarian.

'Of course, Brenda. What is it?' he said.

'Well, you know when those detectives came the other day, they asked if I'd mentioned it to anyone else . . .'

Warton got this at about five, and he slowly nodded, seeing the thing begin to add up.

'Where is Mooney?' he said.

'She left the Citizens' Advice Bureau five minutes ago, sir. We'd left a call for her there.'

'Did she get it?'

'Yes, they told her ... It's apparently her busy day. She's hopping about, phoning in – evidently quite normal. She's keeping her appointments in some funny sort of way, though.'

'All right. Put a car on her. I'll be here,' Warton said grimly.

He wasn't, though. He was at the Yard when Summers finally pinned Mooney. This was at 7 p.m.

'Kicking up a bit, sir. Picked her up at her door,' he told Warton. 'She apparently wants to go to some party.'

'Okay. Let her.'

'Let her *go*?'

'Yes. See her tomorrow. Ten.'

'Okay, sir,' Summers said, long-suffering. 'Ten in the *morning*?' he added, to get it right.

'That's it. Good work, Summers. Very nice. Go home,' Warton said, feeling flexible.

He'd had rather a flexible chat. There was a lot of point, he saw, in flexibility.

*

'You didn't answer our calls,' Warton said.

'I was busy. Late stories. Didn't they tell you?'

Rather a besom; and very alert, Warton saw. Something hysterical about the large eyes.

'I understand that,' he said flexibly. 'Still, you must have had an idea what it was about. Not of interest to you?'

'Of great interest, but we've all got our jobs, Superintendent. Tuesday's the big day round at the *Gazette*. And anyway, here we are,' Mooney said gaily.

'Okay. Fire ahead.'

Mooney was confused. 'You wanted to see *me*,' she said.

'Understand you've asked to interview me a couple of times. Give you the precedence. Start interviewing.'

'Well. Well,' Mooney said. 'Have you had any more notes?'

'Yes,' Warton said.

'I see,' Mooney said breathlessly. 'Would you like to say what's in them?'

'No,' Warton said.

He waited, watching her.

Mooney thought she'd never before seen a more unpleasant-looking individual. She'd heard a good deal about him but the actuality was far more menacing. He wasn't so much like a wart-hog as an intelligent rhinoceros, looking cunningly at her, before the moment of charge.

'Well, you've rather taken me by surprise,' she said.

'Okay. Have a breather. Perhaps you'd like to tell me how you came to hear of these notes.'

'I don't think,' Mooney said, her heart banging away, 'that I would.'

'Why's that?'

'Mustn't reveal my sources.'

'If they're criminal ones, you certainly must.'

'Oh, must I?' Mooney said.

'Unless you want to be an accessory. Ought to know that. Journalist. Criminal case.'

'Mr Warton,' Mooney said, with a glad flourish of her note-book, 'are you threatening me?'

'Just explaining the law. Shouldn't be necessary.'

He watched tolerantly as she busily wrote.

'Do I understand you've just officially admitted that you *are* receiving these notes?' she said.

'That's right.'

'Am I the first you've –'

'Yes. All to yourself, time being. Like that?'

'Very much. Unless it's by way of wanting tit for tat.'

'No bargains.'

'May I further ask, at risk of being greedy, if you're ready to say that the notes refer to former residents of Chelsea?'

'Haven't seen anything in the *Globe* about that,' Warton said.

'Are you saying it?'

'Not making any comment whatever,' he said casually.

While casual, he was watching her quite carefully; her chest was rising and falling jerkily.

'Perhaps *you'd* like to say,' he said, 'whether you have any sources other than the young lady at the library.'

In the breathy pause, Mooney said, 'Old Brenda, eh?'

'That's it.'

'Well, it must seem ungracious,' Mooney said, after a while, 'but I can't tell you, Superintendent. Sorry.'

'Have you given the *Globe* anything they haven't printed?'

'Can't tell you that, either.'

'There'd be no objection to your editor knowing you'd told me. It's obvious I wouldn't go and broadcast it.'

'Pretty obvious,' Mooney said. 'You aren't broadcasting much, are you? Perhaps if you had, Mrs Honey wouldn't have been attacked.'

Warton watched her unwinkingly.

'Have you any grounds for believing that?' he said.

'Have you any for believing otherwise?'

'I'll tell you what I believe,' Warton said. 'I believe your only source was that young lady in the library. I believe you did a bit of guesswork there, and your reports ever since have been based on it. Isn't that about the size of it?'

'Read the *Globe*, Superintendent,' Mooney lightly told him.

He didn't get up as she went.

He waited a minute and buzzed through for Summers.

'Get all that?' he said.

'Yes, sir.'

'Knows we had warning on Honey.'

'Could be a flier, sir.'

'Ng. Put a tail on her.'

'Full-time?'

'Have to. Three men, damn it, eight-hour shifts.'

'Her phone, too?'

'Needs permission. Always trouble there. Never mind,' Warton said. 'I'll do that.'

He did that, and saw the reports as they came in, and read the papers, and at seven went home.

But despite the maniac, life was still going on, including that part of it that concerned Denny's possible entry to the world of film. At seven Steve was in The Potters, awaiting Artie with a pint. Artie turned up at a quarter-past, with his briefcase.

'Sorry I'm late. I wanted all the shit straight. Take a look at it,' he said, before nosing into the pint.

The accounts, bound in a maroon folder, were immaculately typed.

'Who did it?'

'A chick.'

'How much?'

'Love,' Artie said.

'Well, it's beautiful.'

'I *tell* you,' Artie said. 'It's fantastic. We're already there, sweetheart. He's going to query the wardrobe. It's the one thing he knows about. That's where we shuffle our feet and ask his advice. Is his partner going to be there?'

'I don't think so. He was seeing him earlier . . . Look, Artie, you know I think he's only humouring us,' Steve said. 'I mean, don't take off if he gives us a straight –'

'I won't take off,' Artie said. 'Quit worrying, Steve. We've gone a long way on sweet eff-ay. It's a great job. I'm high on it today.'

'Well, I hope you're right.'

'Sweetheart, don't doubt.'

Steve was glad to see him out of his sombre mood, anyway, so he didn't voice further doubts. He just went anxiously there and back over the accounts, bracing himself for the encounter with Denny.

Denny, some time earlier, had been bracing himself, too. There had barely been need to discuss it with his partner, Chen. A few words and a few looks had sufficed.

They had discussed it in the office, and then they had discussed some other affairs in the basement, and he had let Chen off the premises, and returned to his books.

When the bell had gone a few minutes later, he thought Chen must have forgotten something.

He went down to the front door and opened it.

But it wasn't Chen.

'Hello?' he said, surprised at seeing his visitor.

'Can I see you for a minute?' the visitor said.

'Well, just now busy,' Denny explained.

'Won't take a moment, honestly. I'm after information.'

'Information?' Denny said, curious.

'*Honestly* only a moment.'

'Okay.'

Denny let the visitor in.

At a few minutes to half-past seven, Steve and Artie crossed the road from The Potters and walked to Blue Stuff.

'Well, here goes,' Steve said, and pressed the bell.

A minute or two later, he pressed it again.

'Is that thing working?' Artie said.

'You can't hear it down here. It only sounds upstairs.'

'He hasn't gone, has he?'

Steve stepped back on the pavement and looked up. The light was shining in the office above.

'No, he hasn't gone.'

Artie rapped on the glass door and tried to peer through.

'Should we try the side door?' he said.

'We could,' Steve said, puzzled. 'Okay.'

They rounded the corner of Larkhall Street to the dustbins, and tried the bell there. Steve put his ear to the door this time, and heard it ringing. There was no other sound, so he banged a couple of times, and rattled the handle, and while doing it, opened the door. He looked at Artie.

'Isn't that supposed to be locked?' Artie said.

Steve didn't say anything. He felt around in the dark passage and switched the light on. 'Denny!' he called up the stairs.

There was no answer, so he started up, Artie following.

He couldn't find the stock-room switch on the landing, but a slit of light was shining from Denny's inner office. He cautiously felt his way to it, and opened the door, and they saw why Denny hadn't answered the bell.

From the long rafter above his desk the chairman seemed to

be attentively watching them. Along with the flights of wild duck and calligraphy Mr Ogden Wu was hanging, by his neck.

One of the more grotesque aspects of him was that his head was in a bag. It was a plastic bag, and his final inhalations had sucked it into a crumpled, but recognizable, mould of his face. A tiny bulge showed the neat nose, a bigger one his tongue, which was evidently out. It wasn't the only grotesque aspect.

Denny had been hoisted aloft by the stock-room's block and tackle. The long end of the nylon cord had been secured to a leg of the desk, which in consequence was raised from the floor; the whole desk slanted at a slight angle as if from a final lurch by the chairman.

'Let's go, Artie,' Steve said, quietly.

They went, in haste, back through the dark stock-room and down the stairs.

'Hold it a minute,' Artie said at the bottom. 'Lock the door. Use your handkerchief.'

Steve looked at him, but he locked the outside door.

'Where's he keep the money?' Artie said.

'Christ, Artie –'

'*Where?*' They were speaking in whispers.

'Well, the basement, but how the hell –'

'A safe in the floor, something like that . . . Let's see.'

They stared at each other a moment, and Steve led the way.

They stepped carefully into the denim-smelling shop, dimly lit by outside lighting, and then down more stairs. It was pitch black at the bottom. Steve felt around, and they entered the large fitting room, and he closed the door and switched on the light.

'Okay,' Artie said. He could see his image in the wall mirror, and Steve's, looking frail and bewildered beside him. He saw the carpet was loose-laid, and raised the edge and peeled it back, revealing a felt underlay, which he pulled up, too. He got out his handkerchief and felt around with it over the floorboards, and almost immediately found the loose one.

There was no safe. A small metal box sat under the loose board, on concrete. Artie picked it out and weighed it in his hand, and tried the lid. It was locked.

'Artie, we can't do this,' Steve said.

'Yes we can,' Artie said, and put the box in his pocket and replaced the board and the underlay and the carpet. 'Okay, scram.'

They were on the way out before Steve came to.

'Jesus – hang on! We've got an appointment with him. He'll have told Chen. We have to get the police.'

Artie licked his lips. 'Not before we've opened this,' he said.

'Have you *flipped*?'

'No. I haven't,' Artie said. 'All we need is the key. Well, he'll have it on him, won't he?'

'Artie –'

Artie was going back up the stairs. After an indecisive moment, Steve followed.

Denny was still hunched and watching them from his end of the rope. His body swung as Artie went through the pockets. A small button-up wallet in the left trouser pocket had the keys. Feeling carefully with his handkerchief, Artie singled out the smallest and in a moment had the cash box open. Inside were half a dozen small packets and some green paper money: hundred-dollar bills. There were five of them.

'Where's all the rest, then?' Artie said.

He looked carefully under the packets. There was no more money. He picked out one of the packets with his handkerchief, and ripped the adhesive tape and sniffed inside. Then he put a finger in and licked the powder on the end.

'Heroin.'

'Oh, Jesus Christ,' Steve said. He was shaking. 'Put all that back, you bloody madman!'

'We'll have the money, anyway,' Artie said, and pocketed it, and repacked the heroin and locked the box.

'What if you're searched with it?'

'Right!' Artie said. He looked around. 'That other room.'

'The *stock-room*?'

'Don't just stand like a tit. Help.'

Steve helped. They taped the five hundred dollars inside the leg of a pair of jeans in a bale on the upper shelves, and replaced the box under the basement floor. Then they called the police.

But it was a mistake, this incident. And it led to many others; although not to Hoppity-Hop. Hoppity-Hop was on the drawing board, anyway.

Three

Hoppity-hoppity,
Hoppity-hoppity,
Hoppity-hoppity,
Hop.

20

A SERGEANT gave Warton a discreet shake at half-past one the next afternoon, and said, 'Sandwiches, sir.'

'Right.' He hadn't been sleeping; he didn't think he had. But as he sat up on the camp bed and saw the chap emptying his full ashtray into the bin, he realized that he had been at the least day-dreaming. 'Garbage,' he said.

'Sir?'

'Where's Chief Inspector Summers?'

'Just got his head down. Not ten minutes ago, sir,' the man said reproachfully.

'Get him.'

Summers came gauntly into the room.

'When was the garbage cleared?' Warton said.

'Garbage?'

'There were two big metal containers – what do they call them, skips – in that street. We checked the dustbins, we didn't check them. Have they been cleared?'

'Well, I –'

'Get on to the sanitation people. Mustn't be destroyed.'

'Oh. You mean –'

'Do it now. And come back here. Also, want the Cumulative. Get it sent in right away.'

The coffee tasted terrible. So did the sandwiches. He knew it must be his mouth. Apart from a couple of visits to Blue Stuff during the night while the search proceeded, he had sat smoking in this room.

There was a light scattering of ash over the desk; the cleaners hadn't been able to get in. He had a look at the photos again as he drank the coffee. Various views of the room, and of the Chinaman; hanging and on the floor; with the bag on and the bag off. He had been chloroformed before the bag had gone on.

His desk was a litter of messy reports that had ceased to mean anything to him. His head thudded distantly. But he was able to concentrate on the Cumulative when it came in, and to note that it was up to date as of noon.

The fellow Chen had left the shop at six-forty. The two young men had found the body soon after seven-forty.

In that hour the Chinaman had been killed, and in that hour their alibis stood up, so he'd had to let them go. He had done it reluctantly, because he didn't like alibis. Innocent people rarely had much in the way of an alibi. But everybody seemed to have one here.

Warton had methodically had every conceivable suspect questioned, though he knew the person he wanted could only be the one who had sent the O.W. message; which meant one privy to Brenda's tale: Giffard or Johnston, Colbert-Greer or Mooney. One of those four.

He had entertained some wild thoughts about Mooney, but he knew now it couldn't be Mooney. Mooney had been at a wine and cheese session of the Chelsea Poetry Society between six and eight; amply attested, apart from being attended by her tail.

Colbert-Greer had been having a drink at six with a colleague, who had then walked part of the way home with him. His irate fellow tenant Mrs Bulstrode was pretty certain he had been moving about in the room above hers at six-thirty. And an Indian student (almost certainly homosexual) said he had visited and remained with him from shortly before seven. There were loopholes here, and Warton liked them; but he didn't suspect Colbert-Greer. The hanging was not the work of a Colbert-Greer.

He looked at the entry on the coloured bloke: JOHNSTON, *Arthur (Artie)*.

He had been visiting a female who had done some secretarial work for him at Putney, three miles away. She attested that he had left her at six-fifteen; which left a full hour before he had turned up at the pub at seven-fifteen. He said he had gone to his own home at Putney to check some work. Nobody had seen him enter the flat. But a bus conductor, same colour, had confirmed that a man of his description had boarded his bus at Putney at a few minutes to seven, and had got off, the full three miles away, outside the pub. That left twenty minutes between the earliest time the shop could have been entered (never mind killing the Chinaman and stringing him up), and the time that Johnston had turned up on a *returning* bus three miles away.

Well, the conductor could have been wrong. There were other negroes with Afro hair styles. Loopholes here, too.

There were no loopholes in Giffard's story, and Warton brooded over the entry: GIFFARD, *Walter Stephen (Steve)*.

Giffard had arrived home from work at six-twenty; which the caretaker had particularly noticed because he had a registered letter for him, and Giffard had asked him for it. He had then had a shower and changed and gone out again, twenty minutes later. He had certainly turned up at the pub fifteen minutes after that, at five minutes to seven. And the journey would have taken him fifteen minutes, unless he'd grabbed a cab. Even with a cab, there was no time for him to go in and do the Chinaman and turn up at the pub when he had.

Warton pondered this. The timing was neat. It was too neat. At the same time he turned over in his mind another question.

There had been no signs of a struggle at either the front or the back door of the shop, or on the stairs. This indicated that the Chinaman had let in the person who had killed him; or that the back door had been left open for him. All these suppositions suggested somebody close to the business.

Warton also pondered another matter: the absence of the chloroform. He knew now where the chloroform had come from. Inquiries after the attack on Honey revealed that a bottle was missing from a laboratory at Chelsea College.

Among recent visitors to the laboratory were Mary Mooney (who had done a diary item on it), and the golden threesome now under review. This shower had toured the place with a view to using it in their horrible film.

Wherever he turned, Warton found this golden threesome.

A further puzzle was the mode of administering chloroform. A person wasn't given a bottle and asked to sniff. The stuff must have been presented on a pad, as it had been to Honey. Where was the pad, and where was the bottle?

In his bones, Warton knew that one or both of these young

bastards had done for the Chinaman. What had they done with the pad and the bottle?

He had had them searched immediately, and also the premises. But when squad cars had brought in first Chen and then the shop's two full-time employees, Stanley Barrow and Wendy Lawrence, he had been presented with another reason for search. The young chap Barrow had confidentially told him that Wu kept large sums of dollars in a cash box in the basement. Persistent eavesdropping had revealed to him that whenever Chen appeared there was a share-out of these dollars.

Chen had naturally denied any knowledge of this; but an immediate search of the basement room had produced the cash box, under the floorboards; the key to it had been found on Wu. The box had been found to contain sixty grams of first-quality heroin, but no money.

Experience, on such occasions, had taught Warton never to watch the find itself, but the expressions of those who were watching it. A very faint frown, instantly removed, had appeared on Chen's face. Stanley Barrow had gaped at the money-less box before looking hard at Chen, and then even harder at Steve Giffard. The girl had simply stared at it with her mouth open. But Giffard and Johnston, Warton saw, hadn't been watching the box at all. They had been watching him.

Yes. They knew. Bloody certainly, they knew. They'd been at the box. So where was the money? And the chloroform and the pad?

The search had produced nothing, though six experienced men had gone to work.

He had kept Giffard and the black till three in the morning, but then he'd had to let them go; and had himself worked on for hours, before taking to the camp bed.

'Okay on the skips, sir,' Summers said, coming in. 'They were removed this morning, but the stuff is intact at the yards. I've got blokes on the way now.'

'Good. Have a cup, Summers.'

'One out there, sir,' Summers said dolefully.

'Bring it in.'

When Summers returned, yet more dolefully, he found

Warton still brooding over the Cumulative. He didn't speak for several minutes.

'There's a bottle of chloroform somewhere, Summers,' he said. 'Not just the small quantity used last night. Biggish job. Being kept somewhere.'

Summers remained silent.

'Also this costume.' Warton had turned back a few pages to the attack on Honey. Her description of the mask and the wig had suggested a professional kit, so inquiries had gone out to all theatrical costumiers. They had turned up one which had supplied the small film company. They hadn't supplied this particular mask. Still: the old threesome again.

'There are three things hidden away,' Warton said. 'There's the chloroform. There's the mask. And there's the material for making up these messages. He's got them somewhere.'

'Search warrants, sir?'

'Have to – although he won't have it at home. All of this lot would go in a quite small package, shopping bag, something like that. Locked up somewhere, where he can get at it.'

'What – railway terminals, lock-up boxes?'

'I think so. We have to regard anything small and light as suspicious. No reason for anybody to leave it. Get cracking on the warrants. We'll do the lot in one sweep.'

'House searches for Giffard and Johnston. Colbert-Greer?'

'Certainly. Could be harbouring stuff.'

'Mooney?'

Warton paused. The girl had been rendered harmless as a reporter, whether she knew it yet or not. And it certainly couldn't be her. Apart from anything else, she'd had a tail solidly following her.

'Well,' he said, 'in the interests of elimination, yes. But when through, take the tail off her. I want the others tailed.'

'All three? Nine men, sir.'

'I know it. See these people are present at their house searches – want everything in order. Afterwards I'll have Giffard and Johnston back here.' He squinted at his watch. 'Two o'clock. I'll take a kip at four. Bring them in any time after six. You look as if you could do with one yourself, Summers.'

'That's right,' Summers said.

'Whenever you can. Sorry about it. Policeman's lot, you know.'

'Not a happy one. Gilbert and Sullivan,' said Summers, prophetically.

21

At two, Steve cut out for lunch. In the night it had occurred to him that Artie's prints were all over the dollar bills, and he was pretty sure the police would be back. He had been on tenter-hooks all morning. The place had been like a madhouse; the murder a great boost for business.

Chen had called in his wife and an extra hand from the ware-house, so that six of them in all were coping. Lunch was being staggered, the six of them dashing out individually for a sand-wich and a cup of coffee; so Steve had had to look lively when Stanley dashed out for his.

He was aware that Stanley had been keeping an eye on him all morning. Despite the crush and the confusion, whenever Steve turned he had met that bulging eye. With Stanley safely out of the way, he had lost no time. He had left a customer try-ing on denim topcoats, explained he was going to get others, and had shot upstairs; and up the ladder.

The police had put everything back where it was; and the object of their search had seemed to be for something bulkier than his. They had felt among the big tied bales, but hadn't taken them apart. Steve identified the bale and the individual pair of jeans and slipped his hand up the trouser leg and found it.

Artie had done this piece of work. The five bills had been spread out in a line, and as Steve ripped off the two lengths of adhesive tape, top and bottom, the whole lot came away in one piece in his hand. In a trice he had folded it double so that the two ends of tape met each other, without sticking further to the money, crumpled the wad into his pocket, and was down the ladder.

He picked up a couple more of the topcoats, and within three minutes was trying them on his customer.

And not a moment too soon; unbelievably, as he squared off the shoulders of the second, he saw in the mirror that Stanley was back. He couldn't possibly have eaten in the time, and he hadn't. He had brought his sandwiches back with him. He was watching Steve as he ate them.

Steve polished off his customer, handed him and his parcelled coat over to Chen for payment, and said that he'd grab a bite himself now.

By five-past two he was in the Markham Arms, where Artie had been waiting since one.

He was very nervous, Steve saw. However, they had made their plans, and Steve passed the money. While he got on with a sandwich and beer, Artie took off to the toilet. When he returned, they left immediately.

Steve returned to the fray and felt Stanley's eye, even more hotly suspicious, on him all afternoon. Artie jumped on a number 22 bus.

He changed from this to a number 19, and then a 137, and a 133. By this time he was miles away, at Streatham Common. He was pretty sure no one was accompanying him, so he got off.

He posted his envelope in a drowsy tree-lined street of suburban houses, just off the common, with not a soul in sight. This was at about four o'clock. He saw from the enamelled plate on the box that the next collection would be at four-thirty. It was still only Thursday, so that by Monday at the latest the letter ought to get anywhere from Land's End to John o'Groats. But it was only going to Liverpool.

There was no time to return home after this, so he went straight to the restaurant, enormously relieved to be free of his burden, and made it by a quarter-past five.

The two men were waiting for him there; plain-clothes men. They took him home and searched him, and then searched the flat, and he tried hard to stop himself trembling, realizing the closeness of the shave.

*

Warton's sweep had been going on since three o'clock. Work on the main London terminals had been started; and as a grace note, Summers had got permission to inspect anything that the leading suspects might have deposited at their banks. As he didn't yet know which were their banks, he was holding this useful permission up his sleeve.

A little later, while Warton slept, some other research proceeded in a landscape of rubbish dumps. A gruesome collection of cotton wool pads, used for miscellaneous purposes, had been isolated from the general refuse. But it was quite an unsullied one that the forensic scientist at last held aloft in his tweezers.

*

Frank had spent the day making notes in the British Museum. He returned to receive his special frisson shortly before five.

Summers had managed a couple of hours' sleep himself by this time, and was among the welcoming party.

'Well, how marvellous,' Frank said, on having the matter explained to him. 'Of course you must ... Quite all right, dear,' he said to the indomitable lady who immediately peered out of her room as they entered the house. 'Friends not foes.'

'Are they going to look at the boiler?' the old lady said.

'Shall we let them – as a special treat?' Frank asked gaily.

'It still isn't right. He hasn't put the door on. He's got to, by law,' the old lady seriously told Summers, whom she rightly took to be the chief of the party. 'He doesn't care about the law, that Indian.'

'Well, they do,' Frank said. 'They care tremendously. They'll make him put it on, don't you worry. They'll torture him till he does.'

'Oh, lor', are you off again?' the old lady said.

'You never know,' Frank said, with a roguish look at the detectives. 'This way, lads.'

Summers and his three men exchanged glances as they followed Frank up the stairs, and then exchanged more on entering the flat. The place was in a colossal mess, the remains of a meal on the table, cushions on the floors, and a heavy odour of curry, together with a fainter one of incense, lingering.

'Not as neat as a pin,' Frank confessed, pursing his lips. 'Never mind. What can I offer you?'

'Just the keys to whatever's locked,' Summers said grimly.

They took an hour and a half over it, and turned up some interesting things. Apart from a select collection of pornography, the materials set aside were a small screw of marijuana, a phial of white powder, and a folio of colour sketches on cartridge paper.

Frank was restive about the marijuana.

'You surely wouldn't make trouble about a scrap of grass,' he said plaintively.

Summers certainly would, but his interest was arrested by the last item. He stopped at one of the sketches.

'What's this?' he said.

'A mask we're using in the film.'

Summers stared at it. Almost certainly the one used in the attack on Mrs Honey.

'Where is it?' he said.

Frank paused. 'I don't know,' he had to admit. 'I just design them, you know. These are specials, and they get them made up. I expect Artie – Mr Johnston – will know.'

*

But Mr Johnston didn't.

He had all the rest of the specials that they'd had made up; they were in three large cardboard boxes. He didn't have this one.

Summers had radioed Warton, and had gone over to Johnston's himself, with the folio.

Fifteen minutes later, Warton appeared, with Mrs Honey.

'Well, *something* like that,' she said uncertainly, and very Welshly, looking at the folio. 'Only it was dark, wasn't et?'

'You'd know the real one if you saw it?' Warton asked.

'Oh, yes. Only this is just a scribble, esn't et?'

Warton got them searching again, and meanwhile questioned Johnston in a corner.

'Why should this one be missing?' he asked again.

'Jesus – it was after four in the morning! People were dressing and undressing. We were dismantling lights and cameras and recording gear. Do you know what it's like after night-shooting?'

'It was used in the night-shooting, was it?'

'I don't even know that. I can't remember.'

'Isn't it on the film?'

'I haven't seen the bloody film!'

Warton got to the bottom of this one, and worked through the possibilities of the missing costume still being at the wharf, or at one of the actors', or at a dozen other places.

The one place it definitely wasn't at was Artie Johnston's.

*

The search at Giffard's produced nothing, and neither did the later interrogation which Warton conducted at Lucan Place. He was particularly interested in Giffard's chat with Wu.

'How much was it you asked him for?'

'Two hundred pounds,' Steve patiently repeated.

'Your mate Johnston expected more.'

'He's more optimistic,' Steve said.

'But two hundred suited you. What – cash, cheque?'

'All welcome.'

'Dollars?' Warton said.

'Very welcome.'

'You didn't ask for dollars?'

'I asked for two hundred pounds.'

'What would that have made in dollars?'

'I don't know. Three or four hundred?'

'You haven't been changing any lately?'

'I'm not sure I've even seen one.'

'They're green,' Warton said. 'Unlike me. I'm not green, Giffard. You didn't know he had dollars on the premises, of course.'

'I'd heard Stanley on the subject.'

'What was your view?'

'I didn't have one.'

Warton stared at him for a full minute.

'Where's your bank?' he said.

'My bank?' Steve blinked. He told him.

Warton jotted it down. 'Any accounts elsewhere?'

'No. I don't even get too much use out of that one.'

Warton lit a cigarette and looked at him through the smoke a bit longer. He took him there and back through the rigmarole. He heard some cock-and-bull story of the Chinaman having offered him a partnership together with a trip to China. He couldn't trip him on it, however, and he couldn't trip him on anything; so he let him go, and sat on smoking, watching the closed door.

It was past nine o'clock, and he was dead beat. But he thought over the results of the day.

The chloroform pad recovered from the refuse was now safely stored, a future exhibit.

The large-scale searches of lock-up boxes had produced nothing of relevance to the case.

The search at Colbert-Greer's had disclosed that he was in legal possession (as a registered addicted person) of his ration of heroin, and in illegal possession of fifteen grams of marijuana, which might come in very useful. The real find had been his sketchbook; with the shadowy drawing of the mask used in the attack on Honey.

For the first time, if he could get a positive identification out of Honey, this definitely linked the golden threesome to the inquiries. It also tended, together with the drugs found, to eliminate Colbert-Greer, since he would hardly leave himself in such a position if he was a culpable party. Still: open mind.

The search at Artie Johnston's had produced information also of interest though negative: the absence of the costume. He was supposed to have it. His not having it attracted attention to him. However, there were multiple interpretations of this, so he kept an open mind here, too.

And he tried to do the same with Giffard. Nothing whatever had been produced from him. The little squirt was clean as a whistle. And as Warton had just heard, he had an answer for everything.

He brooded on this all the way to Sanderstead.

*

He had a première next morning, at ten sharp, in the cramped and tatty viewing room at the film labs. He had Summers with him, and Mrs Honey, and a copy of the script. He read this with a penlight to keep track of what was going on.

The script was a piece of lunacy, but the film version even worse. He had arranged with the projectionist that when he yelled 'Oy!' he wanted him to stop, and he yelled it a good few times while finding his place in the script. The night scenes were scattered through it, in no particular order as far as he could see. On the screen, scene 186 was followed by scene 92, and then 301 and 124.

But he got the hang of it. Each fresh piece of rubbish was preceded by someone holding up a slate with a number chalked on it, and then smartly clapping the two parts of the hinged board together. And he saw soon enough what the geniuses were up to.

A girl dressed as a Mother Superior was in the first scene, filmed from different angles and distances, pointing imperiously. In the script it said: *Silent action. Superimpose Caption style No. 3: 'I beg you will leave immediately!'*

But the girl on the screen was obviously not mouthing this. She was obviously mouthing a two-word obscenity. She was mouthing it, as the next series of shots showed, to a young woman with a baby who had to reply, *'Mother I humbly obey!'* But she wasn't saying this, either. She was obviously responding with a three-word obscenity.

Yes; very comical.

The young woman had to scurry to the river bank with the baby. An old-time toff in topper was on the river bank. There were a few close-ups with eyebrow-raising and long looks. Then bafflingly, there was a crowd scene, with comical bobbies strolling.

'That's et!' Mrs Honey said.

'Oy!' Warton called.

The film flickered to a halt.

'No, before. Et esn't there now.'

'Go back!' Warton bawled. 'Do it in slow motion.'

After a faint hail, and a whirring, they were back with the toff and his eyebrows, and the board slowly clicking to, and bobbies articulating like marionettes.

'That's et!'

After a minute or two they'd got it, and held it. The thing was seen in mid-distance and between two sets of shoulders.

There were two other views of it, one less clear but showing, interestingly, that it was worn by a woman.

During the remaining nonsense, the toff strangled the young mother and threw the baby in the river while the bobbies continued strolling.

They ran through the whole thing a few times more, and it was noon before they were through.

'Prints of those shots,' Warton said.

*

By noon, Mr Chen had completed what he had to do. He had been very gravely worried at the prospect, but his wife had convinced him that it was right.

He had cut out the required words from the newspaper, but there was one he couldn't find, so he had written it in with a new fibre-tipped pen, and had then thrown the pen away. He had seen how the police had gone about fingerprinting everything, so he was very careful with his handkerchief.

Despite his wife's reassurance, he knew that the police would know from whom it had come. But he knew they couldn't prove it.

And he had a duty to Wu. He posted it.

*

It was the second Saturday in a row that Warton and Summers had worked. They looked together at the sheet of airmail paper and the words stuck on it. One word had been written in with a fibre-tipped pen: $2,500. The complete message ran: FOR CERTAIN THERE WAS $2,500 IN THE BOX.

Warton studied it and looked at Summers.

'Chen, eh?' he said.

133

'Could be, sir.'

'Not a doubt of it. First break, Summers!'

After a discussion with the Yard, and in view of the new policy, the story was given a few hours later to the Sunday Press.

22

By Sunday, Artie and Steve were certain they were being followed, and Artie wondered how far they would follow him. He was up early in the morning, and off to Euston.

His tail had to do some fast work buying himself a platform ticket; but he was on the same train with him to Liverpool. He paid the ticket inspector in the corridor, and took a receipt.

At Liverpool, he was in the next taxi after Artie, and once he'd marked the address, found the nearest phone and rang the Yard in London. The Yard liaised with Liverpool C.I.D. and got him immediate reinforcement, and the tail worked watch and watch with them.

But he was sleeping in his hotel when Artie suddenly took off for London early on Monday evening, so the Liverpool tail found himself en route for Euston, and thus in the same position as the London man on the outward journey. He followed Artie to the Albert Bridge Road, noted the address, and then found a phone and explained himself to the Yard.

The Yard contacted Warton's Incident Room, and in ten minutes the Liverpool man was relieved; and just about in time. Artie and Steve were both leaving.

They had spent a few hilarious minutes in the flat. Steve had a suspicion the place was bugged and had indicated as much to Artie, so they'd communicated what they wanted to say in sign language, and talked of other things for anybody else's possible interest. Artie had needed immediate relief in the bathroom, and found a fresh subject to talk out loud about when he emerged. 'Damn it, I could have brought the old toilet sign you made, "God Bless This Crapper". Remember it?'

'How have you got that?'

'I must have packed it by mistake, couple of years ago. It could go up here.'

'Next time. How were things at home?' Steve said, nodding away.

'Great,' Artie said, giving him a similar nod, and also a thumb and forefinger sign. 'I only slipped in here to say hello. Want to walk me up the road?' He was making a talk-talk sign.

'Sure.' They left together, and immediately they were in the street Steve said, 'What the hell is this two and a half thousand?'

'Christ, you didn't believe that?' Artie said. 'They fed the Press that stuff.'

'Why would they?'

'Who knows? Look, we were there. We *know* what was there.'

'After someone else was there.'

'Why would anyone take two thousand and leave five hundred?'

'That's what I've been wondering,' Steve said.

Artie didn't say anything for a while, then he said, 'Well, screw it. I tell you, it's a put-on. Anyway, there's more immediate things.'

He told Steve some of them. Steve saw him to the bus, and went back home, a bit worried. He didn't like some of what he'd heard. Artie was unpredictable, and rash. The little parcel of dollars could be the source of a lot of trouble.

He worried all the way back home.

His tail walked all the way back behind him.

Artie's tail carried on to Putney.

*

Warton got the reports on all these movements on Tuesday, and also studied the stuff from Liverpool. Artie Johnston hadn't moved much from the parental home. There had been plenty of them in it: mother, father, four other children. The father and one of the sons were dockers. Artie had waited till they'd come home from work on Monday evening before suddenly taking off again for London.

Dollars, Warton thought.

There was many a salt at the docks prepared to swap a dollar or two. The father and brother hadn't been tailed. Only Artie had been tailed; and he had barely stirred.

About twelve, Summers came in with further news.

'Film lab's on the line, sir. Our Artie is trying to bail his film out.'

'For how much?'

'Two hundred pounds. Cash.'

'Hah!' Warton smote the desk. 'I told you, Summers – first real break. Always the weak spot, money. Right. Tell them to hold the film. I'll have him and the money here.'

The blackie was quite a tiger when Warton saw him; had lashed himself into a rare fury. Warton liked this. People in a rage were useful; rash.

'What right you think you got to do this to me?' Artie said. His lips were crinkled and bluish.

'Wanted to congratulate you,' Warton said. 'I hear you're in a position to get your film out now.'

'Screw you and your congratulations,' Artie told him.

'Where's the money from?'

'That's my business.'

'Ten-pound notes, eh?' Warton said, looking at them. 'Didn't have those when I saw you last.'

Artie opened his mouth and closed it.

'How are things in Liverpool?' Warton asked pleasantly.

'None of your fugging concern.'

'Dad in steady work down at the docks?'

'And watch your fugging mouth,' Artie said.

'Watch yours, Johnston,' Summers sternly told him.

'Quite all right, Summers,' Warton said. 'Now, do you want to tell me where it's from, or shall I put a few inquiries forward in Liverpool?'

He already had a few inquiries going forward in Liverpool.

Artie's mouth had crinkled more, and he was opening and shutting it. 'Well – I got it from a friend,' he said.

'Got a name, your friend?'

Artie's mouth opened and closed again. 'Frank,' he blurted at last, wildly.

'What – Colbert-Greer?'

'Only – look – I'd like a word with him first,' Artie said.

'I bet you would,' Warton said, and gave Summers a nod.

Artie waited in another room while Colbert-Greer was brought.

It was Frank's day up among the Pre-Raphaelites in Manresa Road, and he was flustered at the disturbance.

'I understand,' Warton said, 'that you gave Artie Johnston some money – that right?'

'Well, what about it?' Frank said.

'Care to tell me how much?'

'Two hundred pounds.'

Warton blinked.

'Where did you get it?'

'Well – isn't that personal?' Frank said.

'From the bank?'

'No.'

'Give him a cheque?'

'I gave him the money.' He peered. 'Is that it there?'

'I must ask where you got it,' Warton said.

'Must you? Well . . .' Frank said, 'it was from a friend.'

Warton looked curiously at Summers. It was slowly occurring to him that Colbert-Greer's alibi could bear some closer scrutiny.

'What's the name of the friend?' he said.

'Willie.'

'Willie what?'

Frank paused.

'Ricketts,' he said, consideringly.

'Where is he?'

'Well, there you've got me,' Frank said.

'He just gave you two hundred pounds.'

'He sent it.'

'By cheque?'

'You have some kind of hang-up on cheques,' Frank said. 'There's money, you know. That stuff there. He sent it.'

137

'Where from?'

'Well, I don't know where from.'

'Okay, take your time,' Warton said. 'It came by mail, did it? Registered mail?'

Frank thought. 'No. Just the ordinary stuff. In an envelope, you know.'

'Two hundred quid in an envelope. Any letter with it?'

'Oh, yes.' Frank's eyes gleamed a little. 'He said he might send me more later.'

'Why?'

'Well, he owes me it, really.'

'What for?'

Frank paused a while. 'I've got a cottage, you see,' he said, 'in the country. It was my father's. Miles from anywhere. I let him have it for a long time.'

'This is Willie, is it?'

'Yes.'

'Are you saying it's back rent he's paying you?'

'He seemed to regard it in that way.'

Warton looked at Summers and back to Frank.

'Where's the letter?' he said.

'I threw it away.'

'Was there an address on it?'

'He doesn't put addresses,' Frank said.

'Have you heard from him before?'

'Now and again.'

'Well, what was his last address?'

'At my cottage.'

'I see.' Warton exchanged another glance with Summers. 'You didn't look at the postmark?' he said.

'No, I didn't.'

'Not curious at all – two hundred pounds arriving just like that?'

'Well – bucked,' Frank said. 'It was so nice for the film, just now.'

'Yes. Anyone in the house hand you this letter?'

'No. I picked it off the mat. I was first at the post.'

Warton stared at him for some time. 'I expect what happened,' he said, 'is that you just happened to be going out, so you read it in the street, and threw the letter and the envelope away somewhere on the way, and you don't know where.'

'Well, that's it exactly,' Frank said.

'Yes. This Willie. What does he do for a living?'

'Willie. Well, Willie,' Frank said slowly, 'is basically a sort of painter, I would say.'

'And he's going to keep on sending you money, is he?'

'That would be fun,' Frank said. 'But I don't know.'

Minutes later, Summers saw him out, and was immediately back.

'I want that Indian he was with checked out, every second of the way,' Warton said. 'Also test the old girl's memory again. As for bloody Willie – well, try him.'

'Try what?'

'Ng.'

They arrived at a procedure in the end, though.

And Warton let Artie go; though he kept the money.

*

The Indian turned out to have been having a long solitary stroll, without a watch, before arriving at Frank's on the night of Mr Wu's death. On close interrogation, he recalled that it was Frank who had told him the time was a few minutes to seven when he arrived.

The old lady below had said to the detectives who had visited her again, 'There he goes,' when the footsteps sounded above. But the footsteps had proved not to be Frank's but those of a person in the flat next to Frank's.

By five that evening, Frank's alibi was rather shaky, but at five-thirty a detective-sergeant called in to say that an agent in Pimlico had an artist by the name of Wilson Murray Ricketts on his books. The last address the agent had for Ricketts was at Lelant, near St Ives, Cornwall.

He had no phone number for him, so the St Ives police were contacted.

St Ives reported back the following day that the address in Lelant, a remote one, was that of a shed attached to an abandoned tin mine. There was nobody in the shed and they were trying to trace the last occupant.

It took them another whole day to do this, and it was 5 p.m. on Thursday before the local inspector called Warton.

The former occupant of the shed was an artist called Wilson M. Ricketts, now living with another artist, a Belgian. 'Queer as a coot,' the inspector said, 'and very annoyed, sir, I can tell you.' It seemed that W.M. was known as Willie, and he had lived for a period with Colbert-Greer. To show his contempt for him, and while intoxicated, he had sent him £200 as rent, and was infuriated that he should now put the police on him for more. 'He said that in his letter he promised to pay him the wages of a whore. You know, sir,' he apologized, 'we have some funny ones here.'

'Very good. Much obliged to you, Inspector,' Warton said dully. 'And nice work.'

He paused a while after hanging up and looked at Summers, who had been listening with him. 'Well,' he said, 'give him his money back.'

'Still keep the tail on, sir? We're a bit pushed.'

'No, no,' Warton said. 'This never looked like his work. You can take the tail off him. It's Artie or little Steve, Summers, for certain.'

So the tail was taken off Frank, and his money returned; and at six-thirty that Thursday he popped in to *Chez Georges* and gave it back to Artie again.

Artie, rather sombre, was in the kitchen.

*

On Friday morning, Artie reported to the labs, and paid in his £200, and got the film.

They were shamefaced at the labs, but he didn't bother with them. They had to be used, like everything else.

He took the cans, and dropped them in to Steve at Blue Stuff.

Pressure was needed now. Steve would edit what he could of the film. Artie had to organize showings. They needed money, and soon.

Artie thought that money would turn up soon. But he didn't

want the police breathing down his neck when it did. So he worked hard all day; and brooded while he worked. Some aspects of Steve worried him.

Steve was thinking along parallel lines.

Some aspects of Artie worried him. When he got home that evening, he swore.

Artie had brought him the cans, but he hadn't brought the editing gear. This stuff was at Artie's flat: Putney. He was tired, but he immediately phoned Artie and went to the restaurant to get the key.

It wasn't an amicable visit. Albert the chef was limping around swearing in the kitchen, and he gave Steve a burst of passionate French.

'What's that about?' Steve said.

'People in his kitchen. Frank was here yesterday. Screw him. Anyway, don't forget to leave the key under the mat.'

'Okay.'

Steve pushed off to Putney, thoughtfully. No word of apology from Artie at forgetting the gear. But he kept calm. He had work tonight and needed all the freshness he could muster.

He let himself into Artie's flat, and picked up the gear. It was in a box, and as he hefted it off the shelf a folder sticking to the underside fell to the floor, spilling papers.

Steve put the box down and bent to pick them up, and paused. The papers were sheets of sketches and dialogue. A closer inspection showed it was an alternative version of the script.

Alternative ideas for the script had always been discussed.

These ideas hadn't been discussed.

Steve took off presently with the editing gear, leaving the key under the mat, and caught a cab at Putney Bridge.

He thought hard in the cab about what he had just seen.

An hour later, Artie suddenly thought of it, too, and his stomach knotted up.

He'd meant to lock the folder in a drawer. He'd meant to deliver the editing gear himself. He kept making these slips. He remembered that Steve had had to remind him, when they

141

were running from Denny's, that they had an appointment with him. It was Steve who had cautioned that they might be searched. On his own he made too many slips.

He felt engulfed in a huge wave of depression, and wondered how he was going to manage.

It was a late night in the restaurant.

The presence of the tail outside maddened Artie.

It was late, very late, before he finally got to bed, in his back bedroom in Putney. It was actually Saturday morning.

23

THERE'D been a bit of rain in the week which had brought the slugs out, so on Saturday Warton got down to them. They were busy at his wallflowers, so he baited heavily there. He observed a persistent slug turning steadily from the bait. He watched it for a while, and deployed cunning.

Slugs didn't like fingers. Warton gave it a finger. He laid it on the soil, and saw the slug change direction away from it, and did it again, and continued doing it, until the small creature made its own way to the bait.

That was the way of it. He could have crushed it easily. But why should he, when with encouragement the little bastard did the job by itself? Finesse.

'Teddy – phone!' Rose called.

Eh? First Saturday morning he'd had off for three weeks. He made haste to the house and took the phone.

'Okay,' he said after listening, 'coming in. Let Chief Inspector Summers know.'

He hopped out of his gardening togs, and in ten minutes was heading along the Purley Way into town.

Summers, coming only from Clapham, was ahead of him.

He already had the *Oxford* out, and at the right place, alongside the message, on his desk. The message simply said:

> Sing Hey to you –
>   Good day to you.

Warton followed Summers's finger to the full quote:

> Sing 'Hey to you – good day to you' –
> Sing 'Bah to you – ha! ha! to you' –
> Sing 'Booh to you – pooh, pooh to you'.
> *'Patience'*.
> *W. S. Gilbert*.

'Of Gilbert and Sullivan, sir,' Summers informed him.

Warton stared at it. 'A two-liner,' he said. 'It looks hurried. When was it posted?'

'Late last night. So the postman thought, anyway. It was top of the pile when he opened the box, first collection this morning. Street box, back of Putney.'

'W.S.G.,' Warton said, and mused. 'Summers, is the little shit having us on?'

'Which little – Oh.'

'Get his cards.'

The cards on GIFFARD, *Walter Stephen* were brought in, and Warton spent some time studying them. Then he studied those on JOHNSTON, *Arthur* and COLBERT-GREER, *Frank*.

One of the three had sent it. And each one, without question, knew he would be familiar with the initials. He was being had. He was being taunted.

The Liverpool police had provided several fresh entries on Artie. He had a bit of form there; in younger days a tearaway, the odd charge of violence.

Colbert-Greer's cards he knew like the back of his hand, so he didn't bother with them overmuch.

Again he studied Giffard's.

'Well, I'm damned if I know,' he said.

'If it's him, sir, he's playing with us. If it isn't –'

'– he's next on the list.'

'Sailing a bit near the wind – these initials.'

Warton brooded. 'Get him,' he said.

Steve was brought out of a crowded shop.

He was no less collected than when Warton had seen him last, but a trace of strain showed under the cockiness.

Warton watched him carefully.

'Have you run into any trouble lately?' he said.

'Well, I could do without a few of these conversaziones, Chief. Tend to dislocate the day, you know. And the night. Or have you got something else in mind?'

'I'm asking if you're aware of any conflict with a particular individual – personal, professional, emotional. Any reason you might have to suspect anyone of meaning you harm.'

Steve paled; Warton saw it.

'You haven't had one of these messages about me, have you?'

'Why should you think that?'

'Well, I read the papers. If you call me in and – Is that it?'

'That's it,' Warton said. 'Anyone you can think of?'

He saw the young shit thinking.

'No,' Steve said at last.

The colour had drained from him.

'In that case I must offer you protection.'

'What does that mean?'

'An officer will follow you.'

'Uniformed?'

Oh yes; cocky to the last. Warton had seen from the reports that Steve was aware of being followed.

'That's it,' Warton said. 'Wherever you go, he'll go with you. Twenty-four hours a day.'

'Togetherness,' Steve said.

He managed quite a cool smile.

Warton watched the door after he had left.

What the hell, he wondered, was going on here?

*

Steve was sure he'd betrayed no emotion, but he was in a state of some turmoil. He wondered how secure the protection was. He was glad, looking out during the course of the day, to see the copper there.

A different one followed him home, and after a shower and a meal, he put in six solid hours at the editing. The stuff wasn't bad. They had over-compensated at the labs for the under-lighting, so that it looked now flash-lit and grainy. But the green tone would cover it. He saw Abo in the crowd scenes. Abo.

He suddenly remembered that he'd meant to contact Abo. He hadn't by any means given up Abo as a useful contributor. Well, he'd call him tomorrow.

He compared and cut and spliced till two in the morning, and then packed in. He was tempted to take a breath of air to see if his protection was still there, but he knew it would be, and he had a splitting headache, so he went to bed.

He took a short walk in Battersea Park after breakfast on Sunday morning, and the policeman took a stroll behind him. Then he got back to it again.

He was interrupted by calls to the phone out in the hall during the course of the morning. It was Frank and Artie calling to confirm the time for the evening. He didn't know if he was going to be through by eight, but he told them the time still stood. The stuff was looking terrible to him now, and it depressed him. But this was a familiar enough reaction after the long grind. He had put in four hours on Friday night, six on Saturday, and already three by lunchtime on Sunday.

After lunch he took a break and went out to buy sandwiches and beer for the evening, his faithful attendant following; and after a nap huddled again over the viewer. By seven he was dizzy with it, so he stopped and had a drink and put a few records on the player. The sound of Elton John blasting out revived him a bit, and when he returned to the viewer the stuff looked much better. Also there wasn't so much of it left: the final crowd scenes, bobbies strolling. He saw Abo.

Abo. He remembered he'd planned to phone him. It was just gone half-past seven. He had a wash and threw the towel on the bed, and collected himself, and went out to the hall. He wondered where Abo would be. The others would already be on the way.

Artie had been on the way for some time. All day he had been oppressed by the presence of his tail, so he thought he would give him a trot. He was out early, walking from Putney High Street the full length of the New King's Road.

The pubs had opened, and when he got to Stanley Street he thought he'd have one at The Gold Key. With no surprise at all, he saw that within a couple of minutes his tail was in there with him: buying himself a lager-and-lime in the saloon, where he could keep an eye on him across the bar.

Artie chatted a while with the landlord, Logan, and sipped his pint, and presently placed it down. 'Watch that,' he asked him. 'Just going for a leak.'

The tail waited two minutes and went for a leak himself.

The Gents' was empty. He tried the outer door and found it unlocked, and went frantically out. Stanley Street was empty, too. The tail hared round the corner into the King's Road. But Artie wasn't there, either.

*

Steve's first coherent thought, on finding himself safely back on his own side of the door again, with the thing slammed and the chain on, was that he had better get a tourniquet quickly. Blood was simply pouring out of him. With his left hand he felt in his right pocket and took out a handkerchief and got it round the arm, above the elbow. He screwed the handkerchief tight, and looked at the blood still coming out, and heard himself sobbing a little. The blood was all down his shirt and trousers. It had soaked into the carpet by the door.

He could hardly believe it had happened. The students were in the refectory, eating. A few might be drifting back by now, or they might not ... He thought of his protection out at the front. Great protection.

Grills had been fitted to all the windows at the back in the past few weeks, and his bedroom and bathroom were there, so he thought this ought to be all right. The curtains were drawn in his bedroom, and he found the towel on the bed there, and wrapped it round.

After a minute or two he thought he had better get water on it, and went to the bathroom, and ran the cold tap and put his forearm under. The blood swilled away under the jet, streaking his hand and the bowl. He could feel it hurting now, the lips of the wound gaping. He was cut almost to the bone. He had barely felt it before; just a quick keen slice.

He didn't know if it was such a great idea to hold the wrist under water. He could lose an armful of blood. He held the arm up and swathed it round with the towel again, and got another towel, and wrapped that round, too.

He was confused by the noise from the record-player. Elton John was still blasting away. It hadn't occurred to him to turn it down, and he went and did so now, and looked around bewildered. His clips of film were still hanging from the make-shift hooks; the viewer still on. He switched it off, and tried to think what to do. Someone had to turn up soon.

He thought he heard a movement outside. It could be students returning from dinner, but he wasn't sure so he waited, listening, and presently there was a tap on the door.

He said breathily, 'Who is it?'

'It's Frank, Steve.'

It sounded like Frank.

'Are you alone, Frank?'

'Yes.'

'Did you see a policeman as you came in?'

'A what?' Frank said.

'There's a copper out there, Frank. He's either in the garden or on the street. Will you go and get him?'

'Steve – are you all right?' Frank said, after a pause.

'Just go and get him, Frank.'

'All right,' Frank said, in a strange voice, and went.

Steve waited with his arm in the air. The outer towel had begun to turn slowly pink. Now he could feel it; it had really started now. He felt suddenly very sick.

'Steve?'

'Have you got him?'

'I'm here. What's the trouble?' said another voice.

Steve clumsily released the safety catch and opened the door. A huge policeman in a helmet looked curiously in; Frank lankily peering behind him.

'What on earth is it?' Frank said, staring at his enormous towel-wrapped hand, and the bloodstains.

Steve tottered back a few steps and sat down suddenly. 'Get me a glass of water, Frank. I was attacked,' he said to the police-man.

'What – *when*?' the man said.

'Minutes ago.'

'But he's the only one come in,' the policeman said.

'He came in the back,' Steve said.

'It's locked at the back.'

'Okay,' Steve said, and thirstily drank the water Frank brought him. 'That's where he was, anyway. I went out to use the phone, and he was at the back door, at the rear of the hall. I don't know if he was coming or going.'

'You saw him?'

'Oh, well, Christ,' Steve said. 'He had a cape on. He was all wet.'

'It isn't raining out there.'

'Look, hadn't you better go and get some policemen?' Steve said. 'He could still be here.'

The policeman couldn't get any joy out of his walkie-talkie inside, so he went out.

'Shut that door, Frank,' Steve said, 'and lock it.'

Frank did this.

'And the safety catch.'

He did this, too, and said, 'Do you want a drink, Steve?'

'Yes.'

'Christ, so do I,' Frank said.

He poured a couple of Scotches. The constable rapped on the door as he handed Steve his.

'It's open, the back door,' the man said, on admittance.

'Great.'

'What happened?'

'I just – turned and saw him,' Steve said. 'I thought it was some sort of joke. He had this mask on.'

'Stocking mask?'

'No, a *mask*. It was that one of ours, Frank – something like it, anyway. It seemed a bit different. It was all wet, all of him, this sort of cape, and boots. Rubber boots. It's funny how you react.' The drink had worked immediately on him. He felt light-headed. 'You feel crazy, just running. I mean, he didn't do any-thing. I ran, though. I ran like hell.'

'So would I,' Frank said.

'He came after you?' the policeman said.

'When I started running. I mean, I don't know if he would have done. I'd left the door a bit ajar, thank Christ. I got in and closed it, but he was right there, and he pushed it in. I mean, I got the safety catch on, but he whacked down through the gap.'

'With a knife?'

'It wasn't a fairy wand,' Steve said. 'Christ!' He supported the arm. 'Have they got a doctor coming?'

'I told them you were injured,' the policeman said.

'Wow!' Steve said, rocking it a bit. 'It wasn't actually a knife, though,' he added, hissing, after a moment. 'It was something like a little – saw. I think. I only just glimpsed it.'

'Could you give a description of him, like height or build, eyes, anything like that?'

'Maybe,' Steve said. 'After a bit. This thing is going like hell.'

'Okay, leave it for now. Sorry.'

'I wouldn't mind another drink,' Steve said.

'You're awfully pale, Steve,' Frank said. 'Like a sheet. Do you think you'd better?'

'I'll have a drag, then.'

Frank lit him one, and soon afterwards the first police car arrived. Artie arrived at about the same time.

Steve saw his face peering in behind the detectives.

'What happened?' Artie said.

The police checked the house rapidly. The huge Victorian mansion had its four storeys partitioned into thirty-six individual bed-sitters. Most of the rooms were locked, the students still in the refectory. When they had checked lists, and found out who was out, and who should be in, only one room remained to be investigated. It was on the top floor and occupied by a Dutch girl known as Grooters.

The police car hadn't brought a doctor, though one was on the way, so Steve went up with the investigating party.

Grooters had evidently been doing a bit of ironing. The electric iron had been knocked off the table and had burnt a triangle in the carpet. It would have burnt Grooters's head, if it was there, but it wasn't. Instead, it had set frothing and hissing the large bog of blood left by her head. Her head was nowhere in the room.

The girl's plumpish trunk was lying on its front, her black slip raised but her underwear undisturbed. Her fluffy slippers had come off. Large bloody footsteps led to the bathroom, and water was running there; the shower was full on, and so was one of the taps in the hand-basin. In the basin was the head. One of the detectives picked it up. Only one of the blue eyes was closed in a kind of leery bedraggled wink. The man looked at the face for a moment, and put it back in the basin again.

Apart from the two detectives, Steve had been the only one allowed in the room, and hearing the sound coming out of him, one of the detectives quickly hurried him out.

'Not here,' he said urgently. 'Mustn't disturb anything.'

Steve was sick outside on the landing.

When they had got him, white and shaking, downstairs, Summers had arrived. He had not hurried immediately upstairs, but was going through the bursar's list, which the caretaker had supplied. The dead girl had signed herself in, in the Continental manner, surname first, GROOT, which was why she was afterwards nicknamed Grooters. But her full name, he saw, was Wilhelmina Sonje Groot. Yes, W.S.G.

When Warton arrived, twenty minutes later, it was the first thing he wanted to know, too.

24

THE full conference was on Wednesday, three days later. The story was a world one now, and Warton felt himself on trial. He had eaten no breakfast and was pale; and also, Summers thought, dangerous; so he kept his own activities discreet.

'Both psycho reports, sir.'

'*Summaries!* Not reading out that bloody lot.'

'Yes, sir. And cards?'

'Don't want cards. Photos.'

'In, sir. You've got them.'

Warton knew he was snapping, and tried not to. Keep calm, he told himself. His handling couldn't be faulted – not by anyone who knew anything.

He had written himself a brief note with headings, and he needed time to prepare, so he said, 'Okay, Summers. Watch the clock.'

With Summers gone, he lit a cigarette and concentrated on the headings.

Initials theory.
How theory leaked & to whom.
Why early suspects ditched.
Work on Mrs Honey, Wu & Dutch girl.
Why last is key case. Explain girl.

Yes. He marshalled his thoughts. From the Dutch police and local inquiries, he now had a pretty full picture of her.

A loner, almost friendless. Family relationships in Holland not good, accounting for her presence in England. In the last four months her mother had written four times; the girl had replied once.

She had no known intimates, either at the hostel or at school. Rarely went out. Also rarely missed a meal. How the fact that she had missed one that night, together with her evident preparations for going out, suggested that, unusually, she had a date.

He'd tackle the date question later.

Shrink's findings first : how the fellow had surmised, from her Dutch and British medical records, that a girl of this type would almost certainly have one intimate. She was secretive : kept no diary or letters.

Dutch police's efforts at tracing intimate.

At the London end, on possible 'date', briefly recount the policy on the Press, with a nod at the C.C.

The C.C.'s mode of disposing of the crap on his plate had struck Warton as particularly impressive. He had simply called in all media heads and distributed the crap among them. He had outlined the scope of the problem and the need to prevent panic.

He had admitted that notes were being received and regretted his inability to give details on the grounds that imitative ones would foul investigations.

He had said he had no intention of applying for censorship, relying instead on their responsibility; in return for which he would share every scrap of information that would not vitally impede police inquiries.

And this they had done. They had immediately given them Chen's note; and very useful, too, in Warton's view; money a fruitful source of dissension among thieves.

The girl's possible date was an even better story, and it had been widely used. But no date had shown up.

Yes. He continued with the list.

Theories on date.
How girl 'set up'.
Materials cached.
Reasons for lopping (shrink).
Money.
Permissions wanted.

Summers knocked. 'Time, sir.'

'Right.'

He kept calm. He knew he was quite normal.

Summers thought he looked so sick, he wondered if he'd throw up before he got to the car.

Case in hand, all quite normal, Warton went down to the staff car and sat in the rear. 'Okay,' he said.

He saw the fellow looking at him twice.

Just as the car turned into the forecourt of New Scotland Yard, his stomach gave a single heave.

He'd met the Commissioner and the Assistant Commissioner, of course. Bloody full house, though: C.C.; all crime commanders; several chaps of his own rank pulled in from other cases.

But he kept calm. He saw a carafe and glass had been placed ready for him; expected to speak for some time, evidently. Well, he would.

He spoke for over an hour.

After the first ten minutes, he knew it was all right.

He walked through the initials theory. He swung into the theories on the girl's possible 'date'.

If the murder had been planned to take place in the room, and the elaborate preparations indicated that this was the case, the murderer had to ensure that she would be there at a time when everyone else was eating. He would have arranged this time with her; he would have told her not to eat first. He would have 'set her up'.

The preparations had certainly been elaborate. Three keys copied: one to the back door of the hostel, one to the room adjoining the girl's, and one for the partition door between the two rooms. The suspect with easiest access to the keys (which were available and labelled in the caretaker's small room, normally locked) was Steve Giffard; indicating that, he, too, had been set up.

'Just one moment, Ted.' It was Battersby. Warton wasn't put out. Battersby had written the highly esteemed internal reports for the Yard on several complex provincial cases, and Warton respected him. 'You haven't, I'm sure, overlooked the possibility of this Steve "protecting" the culprit – despite the attack on him.'

Warton nodded. 'No, I haven't. You mean an arrangement of some kind between Steve and the murderer, with the attack on him as part of it? Well, if so, I think we can say something went wrong with the arrangement. It needed sixteen stitches. This doesn't mean there wasn't one, of course. It *could* have gone wrong. Or it could have gone sour, with the chap trying to do for Steve to protect himself.

'Possible. I'll explain later why I don't buy it – and the same with the idea of his "protecting" the other guy, that is, by falsifying his account to conceal the chap's identity. Let's just take the attack on him again.'

He gave Steve's account of it: his trip out to the hall, his first glimpse of the dripping figure in mask, cape and boots at the rear door; his dash back to his own room; the small hand-saw type of implement that had sliced through the gap in the doorway.

'There are two interesting points here. First, the weapon wasn't a saw. The forensic evidence shows that the head was

153

severed with a cleaver, Continental type – sharp cutting blade with a round serrated end. Almost certainly he was attacked with the same weapon. We've done some studies. Steve is a smallish chap, just over five foot six. From his angle, and in that light, the end of such a cleaver, if wielded by a chap over half a foot taller does appear as something like a saw.

'Secondly, his description of the figure, and the amount of detail he gives . . . I'm not talking about the cape and boots, of which we knew nothing. We have to take his word on that. But on the mask itself, particularly the neck, his account is identical with Mrs Honey's, even to the differences she noted between the one on the film and the one she saw. If you'll just look at – photo number five . . .'

He had distributed the blow-ups of the film frames.

'. . . you'll see it's quite an elaborate job. It sits on the shoulders, secured at the back. You will notice the long swan-like neck. Well, there was nothing swan-like about the chap who attacked Mrs Honey. She said the neck was short and thick. Steve Giffard told me the same. There's a reason for this,' he said, noting the puzzled frowns coming at him.

He paused and shuffled through the prints.

'Photo three gives a better idea. The wearer is, in fact, a woman, and the mask was designed for her. Colbert-Greer told me she simply had a long neck – so the mask has since evidently been altered. Also that enormous hair style. In a later scene of the film, the girl has to take the thing off. Underneath she has an even bigger hair style. The construction of the mask takes into account this big hair style.'

In the pause the Commissioner said, 'I'm not quite sure, what the implication –'

'The coloured chap, Artie Johnston, has a big hair style. But he also has a man's neck. And that's what's been altered.'

'Ah.'

'So taking it all together, I don't see Steve "protecting" him. Similarly on height. Mrs Honey made a particular point that her attacker was very tall and slim. So did Steve. Artie Johnston is six foot one. I think the chap is giving an entirely accurate account of what he saw. Of course, this doesn't absolve him of collusion – if some strange brand of double-think is going on that we haven't yet figured. However, if there was an arrangement, it's hard to see what his contribution can have been. The keys? Perhaps. The costume? Certainly not.

'We can say without any question that he had no way of hiding the costume. From the moment his rooms were searched after Wu's murder, he has been tailed every moment. There is no way he could suddenly have produced it. Which leaves us with Artie.'

It also left Warton with the embarrassing story of Artie slipping his tail. He told it poker-face, and heard the heavy silence as he did so.

'Where *that* leaves us,' he said, 'is into the problem of where Artie *could* have kept the costume. That is, if it was worn. Again, I've got to repeat, we only have Steve Giffard's word for it. If it was worn, we have to ask why. The answer might be either for shock effect, or for protection. The attack, after all, might not have succeeded. The girl might have escaped, to identify him. But if worn, where was it, and where is it?'

He told of the theories on this front. Artie had carried only a slim note-case when he left home, and had certainly turned up at the hostel carrying just that. His story was that, on slipping his tail, he had gone for a walk.

Their latest thinking was that he might have an extra rented room somewhere, a place chosen for speedy access. A small item had just been fed to the local press: a low profile story that would not be picked up by the London evenings, but that might bring the right landlady forward.

'However, whatever else he's got there, it's very doubtful if he'll have the money.'

Wu's twenty-five hundred dollars, Warton was almost certain, were now in Liverpool. He didn't think Artie had been foolhardy enough to carry the money with him. He thought he had probably posted it, in one or more covers, and had then gone up to make arrangements for what he wanted doing with it.

'But before going into that,' Warton said, 'I'd like to take up what seems to me to be the key aspect. The decapitation. Why he did it. The girl was already dead. He had nothing against her; no reason to mutilate or humiliate her. I made it a priority to get a psychiatric reading of it.'

The reading was from a government expert who had in his care some dozens of psychotic killers 'detained at Her Majesty's pleasure'. He had seen all the evidence, including the notes. His first important finding was that instead of the wild and eccentric individual suggested by the Press, the person they were after was one in a state of over-control.

'Of what?' the Commissioner said.

'He controls himself beyond the limits normal for him. He gets up a head of steam, and when it gives, he goes over the top. He's then apparently capable of acting out the most violent fantasies.'

As he read out the summary, he sensed them picking up the points one by one.

The decapitation was a responsive act: the Press had earlier depicted a systematic and bloodless 'genius'. The beheading was both a refutation of this picture and a testing of himself; its public intention to confound and horrify.

The evidence revealed a 'basically aesthetic individual, fastidious and well-organized', but suffering frustration, and anxious to demonstrate his quality. He was of a type quick to believe that 'people had to be used', and could swiftly still his sense of guilt at the means deemed necessary to use them.

His mockery and flouting of the police was unlikely to be a sudden or solitary outburst. His social deviance might already have shown in some other form in police records. His outward characteristics would almost certainly be describable in such terms as 'generous' or 'reckless'.

'I'll just read his conclusion,' Warton said. 'He says, "The factor qualifying all of the above is, however, undoubtedly his state of over-control. He is unlikely to break down under interrogation, whatever impression he may seek to give. You are after a cunning and imaginative liar."'

There was a lengthy silence when he had finished.

'What's your conclusion, Mr Warton?' the Commissioner said.

'Well, it's not a bad picture,' Warton said. 'With regard to a police record, Artie Johnston is the only one with any form.

What struck me particularly was the question of not breaking up under interrogation. "Whatever impression he may seek to give." '

He scratched his chin and studied the phrase again.

'He gave me a pretty good impression of breaking up over the matter of the two hundred pounds. Yet he knew he was covered – Colbert-Greer had certainly given him the money. So he was playing with us. Which brings me to the main point.'

He tidied his papers and replaced them in the folder.

'One part of the problem, at least, is over. While working on it, it looked to us, naturally, as the main one. Finding him. I suspect the real difficulty is just beginning – how to take him. The beggar has caused tremendous havoc, and he's enjoying it. However, he seems to have got in the way now of pushing his luck. I think, sir,' he said, addressing the Commissioner directly, 'that there is one area where he is vulnerable. It's why I feel bound to ask for some special permissions.'

The permissions as Warton had judged, raised some difficulties, and he sat out the discussion that followed.

'You don't think,' the Commissioner said at last, 'it would be safest to pull him in on suspicion while you continue with the other steps? I could get you substantial help from other forces.'

'No, I don't, sir,' Warton said, putting an immediate stopper on this. He explained again : he wanted the man in the open and in the position of having to take steps himself. When Johnston took the steps, he wanted to react as fast as possible, with no one else in the way.

'Good performance, Ted,' the C.C. said, taking him on one side as the conference broke up. 'I'll try and get you an answer within hours.'

'Within a very few, I hope, sir.'

'It'll have to go to the Director of Public Prosecutions, perhaps up to Home Secretary. Good show, though.'

'Thanks,' Warton said.

He knew it had been good. But he was still troubled, as he went to the car, by the suggestion of other forces. It was an alert, unstable, highly dangerous young criminal he had to take.

He wanted no one else involved in the encounter: no ambiguity of signals.

Rain had begun to gust viciously outside, and he watched the wipers flick there and back, thinking of all that could still go wrong.

25

BLOODY Wednesday again; and rain pelting the windows. It occurred to Mooney, nodding and scowling as she wrote, that she'd rarely felt wearier in her life.

'Knitted bootees, eh?' she said. The clot at the other end was feeding her yet another half-witted scheme for Christmas. She seemed to have dealt with about fifty thousand already. 'Well, I can't guarantee it will go in,' she said, 'but thanks, anyway.'

She hung up just as the office boy flung the last roll of proofs in. The elastic-banded scroll whizzed past her ear and fell in the wastepaper basket.

She could hardly bother with it, but out of old habit reached for the stuff and slipped the rubber band while checking the next item on her list. Fire service.

She picked up the phone and got on with it, straightening out the clammy proof pages as she did so. She saw that Normanby had finally made it this week. He'd been crowded out by the rising star of Bethlehem and its festival of advertising.

NEGLECTED GENIUS: CHELSEA'S
ANGER – LONDON'S SHAME.

Fruity. There was a photo of the house in Glebe Place with diminutive Monty pointing indignantly at it.

While she dealt with the fire service she flapped over the damp pages. *The Week's Weddings*: double spread with blocks in place. Property Notes. *Landladies Warned of 'Artful Lodger'*.

Some solid crud to do with candles and paper decorations was coming out of the fire chief, and she let him go on for a bit, tapping her ballpoint, before realizing what she was reading.

A young single man who hires rooms and rarely uses them may be passing counterfeit money, landladies were warned ...

'Bob,' Mooney said, a bit breathlessly to the fire chief, 'it's actually a bit early for Christmas hazards. May I come back at you nearer the time?'

She put the phone down and pored over the item.

Landladies Warned of 'Artful Lodger'.
A young single man who hires rooms and rarely uses them may be passing counterfeit money, landladies were warned this week. Police say his pattern of behaviour is to pay a deposit, collect the key, and then appear at infrequent intervals. Cheques have also bounced from this 'artful lodger'. For their own protection landladies are advised to look in at their local police stations to check out all such hirings of recent weeks.

Are they now? Mooney thought. In an unfocussed way she'd been groping in that direction herself. So that was the way of it. There was no indication where the story had originated, but she recognized the chief sub's hand in the 'artful lodger'. She took the page up with her to the subs' room.

'Artful lodger, eh?' she said.

'Like it?' Sid said, not looking up.

'You old fun-smith, you. Where's it from, this story?'

'Late phone-in, I expect.'

'I might chase it. Special bouncing cheque offer for Christmas. Have you got the copy?'

'Piss off, love, there's a good girl,' Sid said.

He had his direct-line phone to Dorking lying on the desk, and was rapidly rewriting lines for the stone-hand there.

Mooney located the copy herself: in the late pile, a phone-in, typed in the office, heavily subbed. At the top it said, *Contact Sgt Ackerley, Goshawk Rd.*

Okay, thought Mooney, and descended to her vehicle, beside the advertising department.

A very unpleasant ride through the rain to Goshawk Road, and a flash of her Press card, produced Sergeant Ackerley.

'Morning, Sergeant. We're following up the Landlady Swindler. Anything new there yet?'

'What, are you out with that already?' the man said. He was at his elevenses, and still chewing. 'We only phoned it in yesterday evening.'

'No, not till Friday. Press day today, though. We might just squeeze in a landlady or two.'

'Well, we've got nothing here,' the sergeant said. 'It was Lucan Place asked us to put the story out to local papers – they were a bit pushed there. Why not try them?'

'Okay. Thanks,' Mooney said, and biked off, at a rate of knots, back to the office, having learned all she needed.

Within minutes she was flipping through the back numbers. She found the week of Germaine's death, and turned to the classified ad. pages.

Accommodation (Furnished).

Her heart sank at the sight. The *Gazette* was the landladies' special, and a good twenty column inches of stuff was on offer; and the same every week since. Still, it had to be in the two or three weeks around then.

Not least of the reasons for her present dejection was sheer fatigue. Wertmuller, now only a bad dream, had proved not the last of her disasters. After the search of her flat she had shot up to Fleet Street in a fine fury. The police had given no reason for the search but she'd assumed, recalling Warton's threat, that they were after any unprinted stories for the *Evening Globe*, with whatever other information she might have: a diabolical infringement of Press liberty!

To her surprise, Chris's interest had been strangely guarded. To her still graver confusion, on hearing her offers to reveal more about the notes, he had rummaged on his desk and produced the Famous Residents list.

'You don't mean this?' he said.

Mooney nearly fell off the chair.

'We've been nobbled, love,' Chris told her. 'There's a cease-fire on. They give us what they can, and we keep down the flack. We couldn't even use the railway station stuff.'

'Railway station stuff?'

'Deposit boxes, all over London. Didn't you hear of it?'

'Oh, that,' Mooney said. It was the first time she had.

'Have you really got anything new?'

'Well, I'm working on it, Chris.' Mooney swallowed. 'I have access to a lot, you know. Only I'd be happier with a staff job.'

'I know you would, Mary. And Jack knows. We just can't hire now. Of course, if you *really* get anything – who knows? But you've got some nice bonuses coming.'

'Well, thanks,' Mooney said, numbly absorbing his last 'really', with the related inference that they knew now how she'd fed them the story.

But he'd told her what they knew, which was roughly what she knew; so she'd gone home and had a good cry and three gins.

It was with the second gin, which pulled her together, that she had begun slowly to realize that she knew more than they knew. Brenda hadn't appeared on the list of things they knew.

Except what the devil had Brenda to do with it?

Something, evidently. She recalled that in her interview with Warton, only two things had come from his end: one, his piece of bait about the notes; and two, his probing as to her sources other than Brenda.

He'd questioned Brenda, then. But why?

She was passing the library next day when Brenda skipped out for lunch.

'Well, my goodness,' she said with wonderful surprise. 'That hair of yours is really a knockout.'

'Is it really, Mary? My new bloke says so, too.'

'What's he like?'

'Oh, well, octopuses, wow!' Brenda said, giggling.

She had a gay and chatty lunch with Brenda, and right afterwards called Frank; and went to see him. Frank would tell you anything.

What Frank had told her had sent her away reeling, fairly bow-legged.

The detective's theory had been transmitted, via Brenda, to three people, all of whose flats had been searched (Frank was interested to hear that it was now four).

One of these people had to be the person sending the messages.

161

She was almost frightened to think of what this meant.

Frank had mentioned the costume, too; and her own imagination had supplied the rest.

Costume. Messages. Chloroform. The police had asked about her visit to the laboratory without in any way mentioning chloroform. But Mrs Honey had been chloroformed. Wu had been chloroformed. They had been looking for *chloroform*; and a costume. They had searched her place, and Frank's and Steve's and Artie's. They evidently hadn't found any of it.

But afterwards it had been used on Grooters; so it was still around. Obviously it wasn't around in any of the places searched. It was around in some other place.

How the devil did you start looking for the other place?

It was at about this time that the colossal mental fatigue had set in with Mooney.

The 'artful lodger' story had shown her that others were working on it. But the idea had been dawning on her, anyway.

Racing rapidly through the Classifieds now, she realized she was slightly ahead of the field. For one thing the story had not yet appeared; it wouldn't appear till Friday. Apart from the police, she was the only one who realized its significance. And she was also one up on the police. Almost certainly they would already have contacted all advertisers who had given addresses and phone numbers. That left box numbers. Perhaps, as well as feeding the Press this innocent story, they were also trying box numbers. If the police hadn't yet contacted the newspaper to find out the names of advertisers with box numbers, it must be because they didn't want the newspaper, or any other newspaper, alerted.

Mooney closed the file and went below to Advertising.

A nice girl called Pru with straight hair and brown eyes ran the box number department. 'Hello, Mary,' said this young lady.

'Now, Pru,' said Mooney, 'we all know how clever you are, and all you have to do is show me how clever you are with box numbers. The management wants everyone to know what a terrific pull they have.'

'Easy,' Pru said, and showed Mooney all about box numbers. She showed her the file and the cards with all the names and addresses of the people who had box numbers, and Mooney thanked her and worked late that night. Everyone had gone before she moved her bike from outside the advertising department.

26

AT three in the afternoon Warton got his answer and immediately yelled for Summers. 'Right! Immunity for Chen – let's go.'

They went to Wembley where Mr Chen, under surveillance for some hours, was in his warehouse.

Mr Chen came with rimless spectacles and a mild manner, and showed no surprise at the visit.

'It's about Mr Wu,' Warton said, 'and the message we received with regard to a sum of dollars he had. You'll have read about it, I expect.'

Mr Chen said he had.

'Delicate situation, as we all know. However, our only concern is to find Wu's murderer. If it's possible for you to help, I'm sure you'd want to?'

Mr Chen said that if it was possible he certainly would.

'It has been officially decided,' Warton told him, 'to make no inquiries at all into any of Mr Wu's other transactions. If any turn up, during our work, we can absolutely promise we won't pursue them. Understand me, Mr Chen?'

'Understand,' Chen said.

'It's the murderer we want. And any money that was taken. Because whoever took it probably murdered him. Anything you can tell me about that, Mr Chen?'

Mr Chen looked at his hands.

'As to money in basement –'

'You know nothing about it. Know that,' Warton said.

'Exactly. However, in business, quite normal to keep dollars. Often needed.'

'What denominations?'

'Ah?' Mr Chen said.

Summers coughed. They'd already agreed to split the job between them. 'What we wondered,' he said, having received a nod from Warton, 'was whether, in going through his papers, you'd seen any reference to the money. The amount of it, and the actual value of the bills.'

Mr Chen continued gazing tranquilly at them.

'Because if a largeish sum was involved,' Summers proceeded steadily, 'and if, for convenience, Mr Wu had kept it in large bills, the numbers might run consecutively. Any information on the numbers would be a big help in tracing them.'

'Or,' Warton said, 'would also be a big help to know the numbers on either side – if for any reason there had originally been a much larger sum that had been split.'

Mr Chen's nose wrinkled very slightly.

'Rike some tea?' he said.

They said they would.

Mr Chen picked up a housephone and ordered some, in Chinese. His instructions seemed lengthy for the supply of three cups of tea, but he put the phone down presently.

'Tellible business,' he said.

'Yes. Any idea how we could get this information, Mr Chen?'

'Thinking,' Mr Chen said.

The tea came almost immediately, brought by a young Chinese. Chen had a few words with him as he handed it round, and the young man went.

'Hope you rike tea,' Chen said.

Warton and Summers didn't like it. There was no milk or sugar in it. However, they sipped it.

Mr Chen sipped his.

'No, Wu kept no information rike that,' he said, having evidently thought sufficiently. 'However, I know he kept only hundled dollar bills.'

'Are you sure of that – all in hundreds?'

'Oh, yes,' Mr Chen said. 'And new ones. Large sum in new one hundled dollar bills – plobably consecutive?'

'Yes. How many are we thinking of?'

'Twenty-five,' Mr Chen said, adding gently, 'should think.'

'Would be very useful, of course, to have the numbers of any – adjacent bills. Realize the difficulties. Though none from our end,' Warton said significantly.

'Understand. Tly.'

'Yes, well, he's got rid of his,' Warton said as they returned to the car. 'Point of that phone chat – to see if any still around. He'd help if he could. Still – it's something, Summers. On to the next step now.'

The next step, because less private, had all day been generating difficulties at the Yard. But after several hours Warton managed to get a form of words agreed, and Information Room put them out.

The agreed form was that the police now had details on twenty-five numbered bills of a hundred dollars each, stolen in the course of murder from Blue Stuff. All currency dealers and exchanges were being advised. It was unofficially understood that no action would be taken against 'informal' dealers who came forward, and nor would the money be confiscated. The police interest was in murder, not possible currency offences.

'Should freeze the stuff, anyway,' Warton said. 'Nobody will come forward, of course. But if he's changed any, he'll soon be getting aggro. We don't let him out of view now. Mason in place?'

*

Mason had been in place since eight o'clock, when he took over the late shift. It was now some time after nine, and he was jiggling his drink as he kept an eye on Artie, and on the sodomites who were dancing all about.

He was in the gay club, Shaft.

The interior of Shaft was a sultry red from the paper moon lanterns, but the dance floor was a swirling mass of stripes from the psychedelic slides in the reflectors. The place smelt like a barber's and was very hot; also fairly exploding now to the thud of hard rock. Though early in the evening, it was already pretty full, and Mason was glad of Artie's hair style, which meant he could keep him in view without sticking close.

He did move a bit closer, though, discreetly elbowing his way, as Artie moved. Artie was gesticulating at the lights to the manager; a respectable elderly poof, face well preserved behind black executive glasses, except that it was powdered and rouged.

As Artie stopped, Mason stopped, and saw from his watch that it was a quarter-past. He casually transferred his glass to his left hand and with the right felt in his trouser pocket and pressed the beeper there. He kept hold of the instrument, which was switched to 'silent' and awaited the single answering pulse. His partner outside was watching the fire escape and the rear exit. Mason's job was the interior and the front exit; neither presenting any difficulties. The enormous first-storey club-room was approached by a single flight of stairs with a wicket gate at the top; two burly bouncers carefully examined membership cards and photographs there.

Mason's credentials had been in order (though quite new and obtained rapidly through special channels, despite the club's long waiting list).

He got the answering pulse and removed his hand.

'May I buy you a drink?'

An eager young fag, very pert in urchin cut and ear-rings, had accosted him.

'Got one, thanks,' Mason said, showing it. 'Just waiting for a friend.'

'Sorry,' said the young fag politely.

Quite. They were terribly polite here. After his first, acclimatization, shock, Mason had seen that. He'd thought he might feel like hitting the first one who propositioned him, but he hadn't felt like that at all. They were so polite, and all terribly nice; 'gay' the word. There was a sensation of excited gaiety in the air, not so much of abandon as of release, as if pressures were lifted and they could be what they wanted to be. What they seemed to want to be was gay and dressed-up. Eyes shone all around.

Artie seemed to have become stuck in a long and contentious discussion with the manager, who was worriedly shaking his head, one finger on long upper lip; so Mason settled on his heels and looked about him.

Five or six hundred people were in the huge murky barn of a place, a hundred or so on the dance floor, others chatting around or lounging on banquettes. A line of young male prostitutes fringed the dance floor, braceleted hands clicking, slim hips jiggling. There was a sprinkling of lesbians about. One, very dramatic in sombrero and high boots, was threading her way through the crowds, casting long looks. Another stood immediately in front of Mason, handsome in black velvet cloak and pearls; except that when she turned, Mason saw it was a man, quite beautiful with green eye-liner and silvery evening purse.

Mason gave him a smile, and received in return a haughty toss of the head and, presently, a backward puff of smoke from a long cigarette holder. But he had to move again. Artie was moving; up the couple of broad steps that led to the lounge and dining area.

Tables were spread here, and banquettes grouped as pews for greater intimacy. A little necking seemed to be going on, but not much, the prevailing atmosphere almost of marital propriety; partners' hair being smoothed, collars adjusted. A grave young couple, both mandarin-moustached, quietly sat and held hands as they drank in one pew. In another a raffish threesome sprawled; one of them, high safari boot cocked on a table, for all the world like a dissolute young buck just in from hunting.

Mason saw Frank suddenly. He was with his Indian friend. He also saw that Artie had seen Frank; and that Frank had seen Artie. After the briefest of glances, they turned away.

Hello-hello, thought Mason . . . But he had to stick to Artie, who was now moving well out of range of Frank. He was moving to the buffet table. Some further argument seemed to develop over the buffet table, and Artie and the manager disappeared into the latter's office.

There were no problems with this office: only one door to it, as Mason knew. He had studied the layout. He kept it in view, however, and when Artie reappeared followed him again.

He hung around in the club till a little after eleven, when Artie left. He had been keeping up the quarter-hour sequence of signals, and he gave the double one now, and on his way to the door received the double answering pulse that meant his partner was making his way to the front.

He gave Artie a couple of minutes and went out himself.

The unmarked police car was already on the corner of the street.

'On foot,' his partner said. 'Turned into the King's Road.'

Mason turned into the King's Road, too; and when Artie picked up a cab, himself got into the trailing police car.

By half-past eleven, Artie was home and Mason in position at the front of the house, his partner at the rear.

They stayed there till half-past three, when they were relieved and driven back to Lucan Place. Mason made his report there in the Incident Room, and then was driven home; and on the way back remembered he'd forgotten to mention Frank.

He was so tired he couldn't think if the incident, or non-incident, was important or not. But tomorrow was another day; except that it was already here.

27

ARTIE was up early in the morning. He briskly made breakfast, picked up the newspaper, and glanced at it while eating. Unemployment figures terrible, inflation rate terrible; everything fugging terrible. But he suddenly saw something worse, and stopped eating.

He read the story several times. They had the *numbers*?

His first thought was to call Liverpool right away.

There was no phone at home, but he knew how he could get his father at the docks. Then he knew he couldn't. Every time he picked up the phone lately there was a click.

For the same reason, he couldn't send a telegram. Or an express letter.

He read the thing a couple of times more.

It was a put-on, he knew. But they wouldn't know at home that it was a put-on. He wondered if he should ring from a box.

It would take time to get the old man; and maybe they tapped boxes, too . . . Perhaps he should get Steve to ring. But he hadn't figured yet how much to tell Steve.

Hot shit!

He couldn't eat any more breakfast. He couldn't even drink coffee. He lit a cigarette and blinked the smoke out of his eyes and cleared and washed the breakfast things.

He had a lot of calculating to do, and he sat and did it for an hour until he could call Isaacs, the new guy putting money into the film. Isaacs was a small-time distributor, and on the basis of the rough-cut, Artie had wrung £500 out of him.

He heard the phone click as he picked it up, and mouthed a silent obscenity into it. But he got Isaacs and told him the problem that had arisen at Shaft.

'So what do you want, Artie? I'm not a caterer.'

'Just another hundred quid,' Artie said.

He managed to screw Isaacs up to fifty, and called Steve.

'Did you fix Shaft?' Steve said.

'No problem. When can I see you?'

'I've got therapy at twelve. Say – two o'clock?'

'Okay.'

'Listen, what the hell is this in the paper about –'

'At two, then,' Artie said. 'I'm pushed, Steve.'

He hung up, sweating.

He knew he ought to call Frank on the problem at Shaft, but he didn't call him. There were one or two ideas he wanted to feed Steve, and he didn't want Frank there.

He made some other calls, and also some black coffee, and carried on with the paper work, and by two was at Steve's.

Steve's arm was in a sling. There was a double layer of sutures in the wrist, and he was moodily nursing it as he opened the door.

'Is it hurting?' Artie said.

'It's okay. Just this Bitch of Buchenwald who does the therapy . . . What's this with the money?'

Artie made silent inquiries as to bugging.

'No, that's over,' Steve said.

Artie put the record-player on, all the same. 'I already told you,' he said, when he'd done so, and at high volume. 'It's a fugging put-on.'

'But – twenty-five hundred dollars, and they know the numbers?'

'They know nothing,' Artie said.

'But *what* twenty-five hundred dollars? It's that sum again.'

'Yeah.' Artie paused. Time to go to work now. 'Well, I've been thinking about that,' he said. 'You know you said someone must have been there before us – well, I mean, shit, someone obviously was. But maybe there was another two thousand there.'

'Well, that's what –'

'Forget the Press. That's bananas. If they knew the numbers would they keep them secret? They don't know them – point one. Point two, if the police information is correct, where would they have got it from?'

Steve thought.

'Stanley?' he said.

'How, Stanley? If Stanley knew so well, they'd have nabbed him. Who else *must* have known, for certain?'

'Chen?'

'Chen ... And with him, it's got to be right. I mean, if he took the money himself, he wouldn't have told them, would he? So if he *knew* Denny had twenty-five hundred dollars when he left, and we found only five hundred, then someone definitely took two thousand. Right?'

'Right,' Steve said.

'Yeah. Whose idea was it to ask Denny for money in the first place?'

Steve looked at him.

'Have you flipped again?' he said quietly.

'No. I've just been thinking about it.'

'Well, skip it.'

'Okay. Another point,' Artie said. 'Who turned up first after, you know, that poor Dutch chick?'

'We'll drop it now,' Steve said.

'No, we won't. We'll get it out of the way,' Artie said. 'I mean,

170

Christ, I don't even know what you're thinking. You couldn't think it was me, could you?'

'Oh, well, Jesus Christ, Artie –'

Artie saw Steve was embarrassed and not looking at him.

He threw in his final effort.

He said, 'Steve, do you honestly think – I mean, could you imagine me attacking *you,* in any circumstances?'

'Artie, I'm not listening any more. It's finished. Over,' Steve said.

'Well I said it now,' Artie said. 'But just before we finish with it, I want you to do something for me.' He threw just about everything into this. 'You're sure you're not being followed any more?'

'Certain.'

'Then call this number.' He had written it on a cigarette. 'Ask for Horace Johnston – it's my old man. Do it before five. You might have to hang on some time. When you get him, say you're speaking for Artie. Don't say who you are – just you're speaking for Artie. Tell him not to believe what he reads, but that Knocker better hang on to what he's got.'

'Knocker?'

'Just that. And don't phone from here. Do it from a box. Have you got enough coins? Here's some coins. Have you got the message?'

'He shouldn't believe what he reads, and Knocker better hang on to it.'

'Right. And when you're through, smoke that cigarette. Don't forget. I don't want you involved, Steve.'

'Okay,' Steve said. 'Now – Shaft.'

'Shaft,' Artie said with relief, and went into the couple of snags they'd got there.

He explained the chief poof's reluctance to have higher wattage in his reflectors, and the difficulty that had arisen with the food. They apparently put out a hundred quid's worth of food on the big buffet table, and the old man didn't want to lay it out early in the day, when they would be shooting with their own extras, because it would stale by evening. He had no objection to dressing the table for them, et cetera . . .

'I half fixed that,' Artie said, and told of the extra fifty quid he'd wrung out of Isaacs. 'It's really up to you what you want there. I thought we could finalize it, with the camera angles, on Sunday.'

'With Frank,' Steve said.

'Okay.'

They went through ideas for the new lighting plan that would be needed and the relevant script pages, while Artie pondered how to settle the next outstanding matter. He said, 'See, we been pretty tied up the last few weeks. I had some other ideas how the end should go. I jotted them down on paper, actually.'

'Oh, yes?' Steve said.

'I thought once we'd got Shaft and the Lucan pub and the other interiors out of the way we could have a full discussion. It doesn't affect what we shot. It's just – a different conception.'

'Well, let's do it,' Steve said.

'Sure.'

'All of us. Including Frank.'

'Sure,' Artie said again.

He wasn't so tense when he left.

He thought it had gone not too badly.

He still had a lot to do when he got back. He talked the wardrobe people into accepting a hundred on account, ironed out the wrinkles with the leading actors they'd be needing, and at five blinked his way out of the role of producer back to that of part-time waiter.

He bussed his way down the King's Road to *Chez Georges* to walk right into a new problem.

Serge had the 'flu, and Georges had a special gourmet lunch booked for the following day.

'Oh, Christ, Georges, I've got a lot on tomorrow,' Artie said.

There was equipment-hire as well as wardrobes, both needing deposits, and both to be talked into a couple of things they didn't yet know about; and gourmet lunches went on till four. That left barely a couple of hours before the evening session.

'Artie, I'm relying on you. I'm not well myself,' Georges

pleaded with him in French. 'And Albert is in a terrible mood. Do me this favour.'

It was true Georges wasn't looking well himself; and Albert lately always in a terrible mood; so Artie saw he'd have to do it, and worked tensely through the evening, all the strain suddenly returning.

He wondered if Steve had got through to the old man, or if there'd been some mess-up; if perhaps Steve was still being followed without knowing it. He knew he was being followed himself; two of the pigs out there, at back and front.

At midnight he had a stand-up row with Albert, after doing the Ansafone orders; the chef, hopping imperiously on his short leg, abruptly ordering him to be there at nine sharp in the morning to help prepare the gourmet special. Georges had to come down to the bar and make peace with a cognac all round; but Artie was still smouldering when he left.

Thursday was not a late night at the restaurant. It was before one when he left; the two pigs still in attendance, of course.

*

On Friday morning, Artie thought Albert could screw himself, and he didn't turn up till ten. He found the chef in the downstairs store-room, fairly dancing with rage. However, his late arrival seemed to be no part of it. Albert was waving a letter. He had managed to pick his way through a portion of it, but could scarcely believe what he read.

Artie read it for him. The letter was from the Marlborough Street Magistrates' Court, and addressed to Mr Albert A. Marigny. It said Albert, being a driver of a vehicle, had unlawfully caused such vehicle to be parked contrary to Regulation 6 of Section 46 of the Road Traffic Act, and in addition he hadn't produced his driving licence.

Albert nearly blew his mind. He said of course he hadn't produced the licence. It had been in his wallet which had been stolen, together with his jacket, from this same car. Were they all mad in this arse-hole of a country?

Artie told him there must have been a mix-up with the licence, but they'd get him for the parking offence.

173

'What offence? I showed the imbecile where the car was parked!' Albert screamed. 'He didn't *know* it was parked there.'

'You shouldn't have done,' Artie said. 'You should have moved it first.'

Albert very nearly had a seizure. He said it was a country full of madmen. He was the victim of a robbery! They wanted to prosecute him for not having what had been stolen from him. It wasn't the only thing that had been stolen. His second-best cleaver was nowhere to be found, the past few days. It was a nation of thieves and imbeciles. And by God, he'd make a stink. Oh, what a stink he'd make! They thought it normal to go about stealing people's wallets and cleavers?

'Okay, pipe down for Christ's sake!' Artie said anxiously. Georges had arrived, and Marc. He could hear them, above. 'We'll fix this, Albert, don't worry.'

He promised to go with Albert to the police station on Sunday morning, the first free time they had, and calmed him down. But it was a morning of disasters, the next one rendering Albert practically paralytic.

The under-chef was having trouble with the electric beater, which Albert looked at for him – to receive a shock that bounced him nearly in the sink.

It took a stiff treble cognac to restore him to speech, and when he got it back he threatened to leave the benighted country within the week. In the end Artie fixing the beater. His varied experience included a smattering of electrics, and he quickly saw that the insulation had broken down, the earth faulty.

The gourmet lunch ended well enough, with handshakes and congratulations all round; but not till four, as Artie had foreseen. He took off like a whirlwind via taxi, bus and tube (pigs sticking close) and managed equipment-hire, film stock and costumiers.

He was back by six. He could scarcely bother to eat, but he sat with the rest and made the motions. He knew he was showing strain, and tried not to. He had a lot on his mind.

All evening he remained like a piano wire, taking the orders and serving the orders; as far as possible staying out of Albert's way.

174

Friday night *was* late. It was almost two before he was driven home; pigs still there and sticking tight.

Well, tough titty, Artie thought.

But for them, not him. He actually managed a weary smile.

Things were okay with him.

28

'BIFFY,' Mooney said.

'*Biffy*? Biffy what?'

'I know it sounds silly, but I can't remember his other name. He just told me this address, and I didn't know if he'd taken it.'

'Well, I don't *think* he's called Biffy,' the old lady said, in some perplexity. She was standing on the doorstep in her carpet slippers. 'His name's Mr Walker. A retired bus inspector, very nice man. He was the one who got the room from the advert.'

'Oh, no, that wouldn't be Biffy. Never mind,' Mooney said, 'and sorry to have troubled you. I'll just try elsewhere.'

She returned to her bike, and crossed that one off the list. She wasn't doing so marvellously. Wednesday, Thursday and Friday had chewed off nineteen calls (some of them to be revisited: landladies out); and Saturday morning so far had eliminated only another four. It took far longer than expected, and there were still over twenty to go. She saw she wouldn't be doing many today. Still, it could be any one of them.

Next on the list was Mulhouse Street, so she pedalled off to it. It was a nasty morning, damp and raw.

Mulhouse Street, when found, was such a clapped-out disaster area, she almost gave it away. But then she had another think. Disaster areas might be exactly what this customer wanted. All the right qualities on offer: anonymity, incuriosity, tolerance of all peccadilloes short of downright lunacy. She tooled slowly along it, looking for number 56.

Number 56 was almost falling down.

Four barely decipherable names adjoined bell-pushes on the rotting door frame. From her list she saw that the landlady's was Cummings, and after much peering pressed the one most nearly approximating to it.

A few minutes, and another ring, later, the door opened, and a most terrible slut, dead drunk, hung on to it, in her dressing-gown.

'What you want?' she said.

'You were advertising a room,' Mooney said, reeling back at the smell, 'in the *Gazette*, a couple of weeks ago. I wondered if it was still available.'

'No. Went,' the slut said, closing the door.

'Hang on. A friend of mine didn't take it, did he?'

'What name?'

'Biffy.'

'Eh?'

Same routine. Same result. The one who'd taken this one was an elderly widower from Lots Road power station; and God help him, Mooney thought.

The day hadn't begun well. And she had an idea it wasn't the kind that just naturally got better as it went on.

It had started raining again, into the bargain.

*

At Lucan Place the day had started very well.

'Many thanks, Inspector. Much obliged to you,' Warton said, and hung up, face wreathed in smiles, one finger tapping his huge snout. 'Amsterdam. It's sit-downs as does it, Summers. Proved it time and again. Third sit-down, and they got it out of her.'

The police at Leyden (Sonje Groot's home town) had got it out of her mother. After two unsuccessful sessions, she had finally dredged up a recollection of a girl her daughter had sometimes spoken of; she thought she had been at art school with her in Amsterdam. The Amsterdam police had promptly interviewed everyone they could find from Grooters's old class, and they now thought they had identified the girl.

'Introverted young woman. Apparently left the school same time as this poor girl. Went to Munich. Name, Heemskerk –

Nellie. They're in touch with the German police. We'd better do the same.'

'Okay, sir.' Summers took the slip of paper.

'How are the landladies?'

'Coming on.' All of them who had given telephone numbers in their ads had been contacted and called on. The story in the local papers had pulled in three; checked out and all okay. 'Nothing in yet from the box numbers, sir. Still, hardly time yet. I'm sure something will come up there. Good letter.'

'Ng.' Warton was sure of it, too. It was a careful letter, sent from various names and addresses, stamped addressed envelope enclosed for landladies' kind attention in informing the undersigned if room still available; together with cheque for £5 deposit. Most would reply, drawing the addresses, which could then be visited. Those who didn't would either bank or swap the cheque (easily traceable) or tear it up. Few would tear it up. And these, give it a week, could be got at officially through the newspaper advertisement departments.

Warton didn't think it would go a week. He thought he would have his man within the week. In that week he wanted no calls on newspaper advertisement departments; did not want their news departments alerted; did not want this cunning and dangerous young bastard tipped off in any way what they were up to.

They were up to many things, on a broad front, and he looked with satisfaction at the detailed reports of Artie's movements of yesterday. He'd moved around a lot, but not a single moment had gone unreported. Even the time he'd spent in a public lavatory was detailed: four and a half minutes exactly.

'Let him try and send his granny a birthday card, even, and we'll know where he posted it. Last of these messages, anyway, Summers. I'm very satisfied with this.'

'Thank you, sir,' Summers said, gratified. 'I'll pass it on.'

'Okay. Get that telexed off to Munich, then.'

Summers was turning to do this when there was a tap on the door, and one of the Incident Room clerks looked in.

'L.E.B. on the phone, sir,' he said a bit puzzled. 'They want –'

'Who?' Warton said.

'London Electricity Board – Sloane Street branch. They've got an envelope for us. They want to know whether to post it or –'

'What do you mean, an envelope?'

'Addressed to us. Inside one addressed to them. They want –'

'Get it. Right away,' Warton said. 'Both envelopes. Immediately.'

Twenty minutes later he had both.

The outer one, marked *Urgent* was addressed to L.E.B., 147 Sloane Street, S.W.3. It was addressed with one of the L.E.B.'s own printed tabs. The inner one, unopened, was addressed to Murder HQ, Chelsea Police Station.

He and Summers looked silently at them.

'That cunning young sod,' Warton said, 'has thought up a new wriggle. He left this somewhere. Could have been a bus, tube, anything. Someone posted it for him. Well, I'm damned.'

The contents were new, too.

The interior envelope was not the familiar kind; nor was the paper or type style.

There was no type style. It was done in ball-point, in wriggly capitals to disguise the hand, on a bit of blank space in a torn-off newspaper advertisement.

> Hoppity-hoppity,
> Hoppity-hoppity,
> Hoppity-hoppity,
> Hop.

They were so stunned they just gazed at it.

'He might even have done it,' Summers said, 'in that lavatory.'

Warton blankly reached for the *Oxford. Hoppity.*

> Christopher Robin goes
> Hoppity, hoppity,
> Hoppity, hoppity, hop.
> Whenever I tell him
> Politely to stop it, he
> Says he can't possibly stop.
> *'Hoppity'.*
> A. A. Milne.

'A.A.M.,' Warton said at last. 'Well, get the cards.'

In many planning sessions already, they had established that all messages received so far related to people known to Artie – or at least to some mutual connection: Germaine Roberts, Mrs Honey, Ogden Wu, Sonje Groot. There were cards on all these now.

There were no cards initialled A.A.M. The nearest was Mooney, whose forenames were Mary Angelica.

'Couldn't have made a mistake, could he?' Summers said.

'First, if so.'

They tackled it from another angle.

The previous messages had incorporated, however deviously, the mode of attack, or its intention. Germaine had been found in a river 'at even'; Honey had received a 'stolen kiss'; Wu had been positioned to 'dance upon air'; and the planned confusion over W. S. Groot constituted a 'bah! to you'.

They considered what they had got here.

Hoppity-hop.

'Someone with a limp?' Summers suggested.

'Possible . . . Why can't he possibly stop?'

'Shoved under a bus, train?'

'No. Dealing here with something to be done at a distance. Won't do it personally – he can't. Got him covered every inch of the way. Needs someone or something to do it for him. Remote control, like the bloody letter. Hop. Hopping. Jumping. Jerking.'

'Poisoning?' Summers said.

'Could be. Poison, electrocution, booby-trap, something like that. Get the covering envelope out to the Press, anyway. Might raise whoever posted it. Also get me the C.C.,' said Warton gloomily. 'At home. Won't be working today.'

Others were working, however. Mr Albert A. Marigny was. He worried about Marlborough Street Magistrates' Court as he worked, and at the antiquated equipment of the restaurant, and at everything else that was wrong with the place. This abominable country, he thought, would be the end of him.

29

ARTIE was still tired when he woke just before noon on Sunday. He didn't bother shaving, or even washing. He just brushed his teeth and put the kettle on, and picked up the newspapers from outside the door.

They had a photo of an envelope addressed to the L.E.B. The police were anxious that anyone who'd picked it up and posted it should contact Scotland Yard.

Not Lucan Place.

Scotland Yard.

There didn't seem to be a connection between the envelope and Lucan Place. Artie drank his coffee and went carefully through every page of the papers to see if there was any mention of a connection. But there wasn't.

H'm.

He had another cup of coffee and thought about Albert and the visit to the police station this morning. He didn't plan to see Albert this morning. He had a look out of the back window. He couldn't see too well over the scraggly bit of garden or the fence at the rear, but he knew a pig would be there; also at the front.

No. No Albert this morning.

Albert would be hopping mad by now, of course. Well. Patience.

Artie smoked carefully through two cigarettes. A lot of things had to be dovetailed in today, and he didn't feel he had the energy. He had been driving himself too hard. He wondered if he should go on Speed again, but decided against it. When he needed the energy, it would come.

He had Shaft at nine o'clock, with Steve; also Frank. Steve hadn't bought his ideas on Frank. Well, tough titty. It was a question of playing it by ear.

His meal-times had become screwed-up lately. His whole life had become screwed-up. He decided to combine breakfast and lunch and to make it a big one. The next meal after that would be uncertain, anyway.

He made himself a panful of bacon and eggs and fried pota-
toes; followed it with half a can of peaches and two more cups
of coffee, and then cleared up and got down to his figures.

He did this for a couple of hours, and then called the chick
who did the typing for him, and went round to see her. He
went to bed with her for an hour, and when he got up called
Georges. He had planned to call him from here and not his own
place.

This part was going to be tough, he knew. The only other
person with a key was Albert, who opened up the restaurant in
the morning, and he couldn't call Albert. Georges didn't like
parting with his key. On the other hand, he knew Georges
rested all Sunday and didn't like going out.

It took a few minutes of persuasion, but Georges, after all,
owed him a favour, so he knew he would win if he pushed it.
He pushed pretty hard and won.

He took off for Georges's flat in Ebury Street, and got the key,
faithfully promising to re-lock carefully and return it within
half an hour. Then he grabbed a cab and went to the restaurant.

The place stank from the food and the stale cigar smoke of
the previous night. The kitchen stank, and so did the downstairs
bar and the store-room. There was a little hovel off the store-
room, the changing room required by law for everyone who
handled food. Albert came in here, first thing.

Artie did what he had come to do, and then gave himself a
big cognac. He ate a few dinner mints to mask the cognac, and
inside ten minutes was on his way back to Georges with the key.

It was dark now, and he went home and switched the lights
on and drew the curtains. He had work to do with the script,
and he tried to settle to it; but found he couldn't. He was nervy
and restless. He knew the pigs had followed him. It couldn't do
them any good, but he was conscious of the pressure. When
Steve called him at seven, he almost jumped for joy.

Steve had called to suggest that instead of meeting at Shaft,
it would be better if they could talk first at his own place to
finalize matters before getting into a hassle with the chief poof.

'You mean – now?' Artie said.

'Well, the stuff's all over the floor now.' Steve sounded tired.

But he said, 'Yeah, why not? It's giving me a headache, anyway. You'll be here – what, half-past seven? I'll raise Frank, then.'

Artie was glad to be on the move again. His own company, the flat, were giving him the jitters. He caught a bus at Putney Bridge and bussed back up the New King's Road, and made it at Steve's just about by half-past seven.

He saw that Steve was jaded; and the stuff was still all over the floor, scrawled-over script pages and bits of lighting diagrams. He'd been running the film through again, and the room was warm with the weary old celluloid smell that they both knew so well.

'I couldn't raise Frank. We'll have to meet him there, then. Christ, you haven't got an aspirin, have you?'

'I've got some Speed.'

'Stuff that. Artie – this film is one big heap of crap, I tell you.'

'You're just tired with it. Is that arm playing you up?'

'It's okay,' Steve said.

Artie knew Steve didn't like his asking about the arm, so he just made coffee while Steve scrambled the papers into order, and they worked out the line of attack on Shaft.

Steve dictated the list of extra points that had been bugging him, and Artie wrote them down, and at about a quarter-past eight they left. They managed to pick up a cab in the Albert Bridge Road, and made Shaft by half-past.

The club wasn't open yet, but they were expected, and one of the bouncers let them in. The place looked like hell now; the harsh ceiling lighting on, extractor fans busily whirring last night's climate out of the huge gloomy barn.

The bar boys were re-dressing the long bar; pretty young waiters scurrying there and back from the kitchen to the buffet table; the manager fussing everywhere.

They left him to himself for a while, and walked about judging the angles; but before the club opened at nine, they got to work on him.

He showed them what fifty quid's worth of food looked like, and they worked out how to pile it at one end, and track in over the top. But he was adamant over the wattage in the dance floor reflectors.

'My dear, you'll ruin them. You'll burn them out! Surely you can hang your own lights over the top. I mean, I wouldn't have *any* objection to that.'

Steve was fussed by this, and by the non-appearance of Frank, whose technical field this was; so they left it, and went on to other problems.

Soon after nine, the ceiling lights were dimmed and a dribble of members began to arrive. By half-past they were flooding in; the amplification system pounding out the rock.

'Where the hell is Frank?' Steve said. 'He knew he had to get here while we could still talk. Every poof in town is screaming here now.'

Artie smiled a little to himself. He had recognized one particular poof who had evidently had to wait for the crowd to appear to provide him with cover; a cleft-chinned, long-haired poof; his tail.

Frank turned up a few minutes later – happily stoned out of his mind, Artie saw. He was with his Indian friend.

'Frank, you stupid bastard!' Steve said angrily.

Artie discreetly separated himself, and looked away, and was in time to catch a most curious expression of consternation coming at him from his tail. This tail had been joined by another man, and they were both staring at him. They exchanged a few words and the other one left. Artie watched him threading his way out.

The man who had left jostled his way down the stairs, past those queuing to get in; followed by the curious glances of the two bouncers. He had got in on a police warrant card.

He jumped into the waiting car, which took off in a hurry and in a few minutes deposited him where he'd come from.

Warton and Summers were there with the murder squad.

*

The photographers were flashing off at the bundle on the ground, and Warton was questioning the caretaker and a third-floor resident, the two who had seen it happen.

The third-floor man said it had sounded like a bundle of

laundry flopping past his window. But the caretaker, who lived at the bottom, and who'd heard it all the way down, said it sounded more like someone jumping or hopping on the fire escape.

There was no conflict as to the time.

It had happened at twenty-past eight.

The dead man was a foreigner, so they'd informed the duty official at his embassy, and presently someone turned up from there. It was from the embassy of Saudi Arabia, for the bundle on the ground was the remains of a young man from those parts, Abdul-Azbig ibn Mohammed.

Warton had gibbered just a little as Summers said, 'A.A.M., sir.'

Four

For every time
  She shouted 'Fire!'
They only answered,
  'Little liar!'

30

ONCE about a thousand years ago, when he'd been a young plain-clothes man, Warton had stood and watched a chap work the three-card trick in Oxford Street.

The man had shown the crowd his three cards, and he'd said, 'All you have to do, folks, is watch my hands and see what happens to the Queen of Spades. Find the lady, and half a dollar wins you a whole one.'

He'd placed the cards face down on a small table and swiftly moved them about, and when he had finished a sporting fellow in the crowd had ventured half a dollar and won a whole one. In succeeding rounds several other sports had ventured half dollars but had not won anything; for the lady hadn't turned up again.

Warton felt like one of those sports. Three cards had been offered to him, and he had put his money on each in turn, and had lost the lot. He knew how the Oxford Street man had done it, but he couldn't see how this one was doing it. He felt now like a man not simply bereft of half dollars, but also of half his wits.

Just about an hour later, he felt the other half go.

A murder was enacted before his eyes then, and he still couldn't say who'd done it.

The official from the embassy had made a few inquiries, and a tiny old Arab turned up presently in the fifth-floor penthouse. He had been Abo's servant. He wept most bitterly and pounded his chest as he sobbed out a long story.

'What's he saying?' Warton said.

'The foolish fellow,' the official explained with a sour smile, 'thinks he will be executed for neglecting his duties. In point of fact, he didn't. Apparently the prince intended having a party, so he sent him out at half-past six and told him not to come back till eleven.'

'Why send him out if he was having a party?'

The official barked a few words and received another long and sobbing story, at which he paused, thoughtfully.

'What was that?' Warton said.

'It was apparently a very private party.'

'Why was he pointing at the mirror – that big wall mirror?'

'I don't think he knows what he is doing,' the official said.

'Well, ask him. Ask him why he was pointing at it.'

The official asked the man why he was pointing at the mirror, and he immediately stopped doing it, as if shot.

'Yes. He doesn't know what he is doing,' the official confirmed.

'I see,' Warton said, and went and had a look at the mirror himself. It was in two bevelled panels.

Several murder squad experts were working in the room, and Warton called one over to look at the mirror. The man felt around with a handkerchief, and opened it; a half of the mirror opened.

There was a room behind it. A camera on wheels was close against the other half of the mirror. A tiny green eye shone on a piece of equipment on a bench, and the expert went over and fiddled a while. 'It's a video recorder, sir,' he said, 'hooked up with the supply to the screen. The trip cut out as the tape ended, but the juice is still on.'

'Is there a tape on it?' Warton said.

'Yes. There's one here.'

'Play it back.'

The expert did, and after some whirring and a click, the screen sprang to life and loudspeakers all around began coughing and laughing. There were four people threshing around on a bed. Warton recognized it as the big divan outside. He stood grimly watching the perverts at it for a few minutes.

'How long is the tape?'

The man peered. 'Short one. Under fifteen minutes, I'd say.'

Several brief sequences flashed on to the screen, the tape having been erased and re-recorded a few times. Warton saw the young Arab enjoying an act of fellatio with another young man when the scene abruptly changed, to show the room empty but brilliantly lit. After a few seconds it blacked out. It didn't black out completely. Undifferentiated shapes moved and the loudspeakers heavily breathed and gasped. Light flooded again as the shapes swung and became two separate individuals. One was the Arab, fully clothed; the other a grotesque figure in mask, cape and boots, struggling with him from the rear.

They struggled over to the divan and the Arab fell on it, the masked figure on top of him. He remained there a full minute, the Arab unmoving beneath him. The room was observable in such detail, Warton could see the clock on the wall: it showed a couple of minutes to eight. Then the masked figure slowly detached itself, keeping one gloved hand over the Arab's face. There was a pad under the hand. The figure felt in the pocket of the cape and produced two elastic bands and a plastic bag. One band was slipped round the Arab's head to keep the pad in position, and then the bag went over the head and was secured by the other elastic band. The figure stepped back panting for a moment and walked directly towards the camera and the tape ended.

There was silence in the room.

'Want it again, sir?' the man said.

'Not just now,' Warton said, and walked into the next room, wondering for a moment if it was a nightmare, and hoping that it was.

*

He saw the sequence a few times more that night and again next day at Lucan Place where a video set had been installed for him. He'd had a few hours' sleep by then. He had also played Find the Lady again. He had done it with the materials supplied by fate for his very own version of the three-card trick; and in the certain knowledge that each would have a cast-iron alibi for eight o'clock.

This had proved to be the case.

Artie Johnston, tailed all day, had been innocently at Giffard's at eight.

Giffard's phone call to him at seven had been monitored and recorded, and his own activities amply accounted for.

Colbert-Greer had turned up at The Gold Key at just about eight and had met his Indian friend and some other perverse friends with whom he had remained until nine-thirty when the whole bunch had drifted over to the homosexual club.

Yes. All covered. As expected.

He went dazedly through the new material in the Cumulative.

There was a summary of the old Arab's statement. He had said he hadn't wanted to go out. His master rarely ate when he was out, so he had coaxed him into eating; he had cut him a chicken sandwich and watched him eat it before he went.

There were the scene-of-murder details, properly annotated with card, photo or exhibit numbers. There was the Polaroid close-up showing how the body had been trussed : head between its legs, and legs doubled, to produce the elliptical shape that had helped the hop-hopping descent. A length of the nylon cord had been left trailing and its end tied into a knot. The knot was frayed, and some fibres from it had been found in the room beside the partially-open window that led to the fire escape.

The fire escape ran down to a yard enclosed by high walls and a door that was double-padlocked from the inside. Whoever had murdered the Arab had not got in that way; he had got in the front way. He had probably simply announced himself on the door mike and had been electrically admitted; which argued that he had been expected, at least known.

The latter point seemed amply met by the fact of the recording. The murderer had been familiar enough with Abo to have known of the video recorder; had probably himself made the recording. The sequence ran for exactly three minutes, and it appeared at the end of a tape. The tape had had to be run back, or forward, to allow this amount of time.

Why? Why the recording at all?

Warton's first thought had been that it constituted yet another 'Bah to you'. But a number of viewings had brought him to different conclusions. Close study of the Arab's legs convinced him that he had not actually been using them. The booted feet of his assailant, seen from the rear, were inconspicuously kicking them, one after the other. The struggle on the divan was also more apparent than real; the Arab unmoving during the course of it.

Warton went over it again and again. From beginning to end of the sequence, he was pretty certain, the fellow had been unconscious, perhaps dead. The recording was a re-staging of something that had already happened.

Why, for God's sake?

In the act of fellatio that preceded it on the tape Abo's partner had been a golden-haired youth even smaller than himself. The figure in the mask and cape was well over a head taller; a figure of approximately six foot one or two. Warton concentrated repeatedly on the few seconds when it turned and walked towards the camera. Exactly as described in all the statements so far: curls piled high on the head, open cupid's mouth gaily smiling, neck very short and thick.

What the devil!

Something was being sold to him here, and not simply a 'Bah to you'. The fellow had already made his point. Some other point was on offer.

Around three o'clock Warton received the pathologist's report, and got the point.

The police surgeon, who had first examined the body, had himself been mildly puzzled at some aspects of it. He had accounted for the low temperature and the rigidity as due to the rawness of the night and the constriction of the bindings.

The pathologist, similarly puzzled, did not come up with any other explanation, but his clinical examination of the dead man's digestive tract immediately suggested one to Warton.

The last food eaten by the subject had been some portions of chicken and bread. The stage of digestion reached at the time of death showed that it had been consumed not more than an hour – probably not more than thirty minutes – earlier.

'Well, I'm damned!' Warton said, and looked up, sunken eyes gleaming. 'Chicken and bread, Summers. Get it?'

'The sandwich.'

'When did he have it?'

'Half an hour before death – wasn't it?'

'What *time*?'

'Well, that little Arab – Oh!'

'Yes. Well, I'm getting old,' Warton said. 'This bugger didn't die at eight. He died at seven! The bloody clock was fixed. That's what we were being sold. Half an hour after sandwich time, which was at –' he flipped back through the Cumulative '– half-past six, this chap was murdered, and then left dangling somehow until ... Now wait a minute!' Warton's small eyes narrowed. His whole head seemed to metamorphose into a single scenting organ. 'Summers – was the shutter up or down when we went in that room?'

Summers thought. 'What shutter?' he said.

'Exactly.' Warton was shuffling through the photos. 'Too true!' he said. View of room towards window; window open; no shutter visible. But a shutter had been visible somewhere. He had seen one. 'Summers – just switch that thing on again.'

Summers switched on the video again and caught Abo having his bit of fellatio. They watched until the scene abruptly changed, and then sat through the murderer's scene. Throughout the scene, a shutter was visible. No window was visible. The shutter was down, covering the window.

'Well, that's got to be it,' Warton said. 'There's his method. He knocks him off at seven or thereabouts. He alters the clock to show it's eight. He stages the thing again for our benefit. Then he resets the clock, fixes the shutter in some way ... Oh, well, damn it, the knot on the end of the rope! The shutter held the knot. He arranged for it to go up over an hour later. Up goes the shutter, out goes the knot, down goes the body. He'd got it perched there, on the top step of the fire escape. Well, I'll be – Is that old Arab still there, Summers?'

'Yes, sir,' Summers said, silently chiming at this Niagara of deduction. 'And I've got blokes there with him,' he added staunchly, to keep his end up.

'Let's get going,' said Warton.

31

AN Arabic expert, not from the Saudi embassy, was now also there. And the old servant, his execution prospects less imminent, was in far better spirits. He gladly showed them the shutter, and the Western wonders that controlled it.

A photo-electric cell normally controlled it. When the sky darkened over Abo's penthouse, the device in the cell lowered the shutter. When the sun again put the stars to flight, the unsleeping device raised it once more.

The device could be over-ridden by a further piece of technology, located in the kitchen, and the old fellow led them briskly to it. To over-ride it, he said, all you had to do was turn this pointer to the sign that said clock; and he deftly prepared to demonstrate until a closer look showed him that it already was on clock. As the dial behind the pointer showed, someone had set it to eight-fifteen on clock.

'All right, don't touch it,' Warton said, and called over one of his men. He had the shutter lowered, and examined the heavier-gauge steel bar at its base. A slight grazing in it corresponded with the position on the floor now marked by a small exhibit flag. The flag marked the spot where the fibres from the knot had been found.

Twenty minutes later, at Lucan Place, he was back at Find the Lady again.

He did it with Summers and three other members of his inner team, one of them, specifically invited, Mason. He had already marked the young fellow for promotion.

The question now was not alibis for eight o'clock, but alibis for seven o'clock, and only one of them showed up as shaky.

He caught Mason coughing a little, and looked at him.

'All I was thinking, sir,' Mason said, pinking a bit, 'is that every time we've been led to a particular bloke, it has turned out not to be that bloke. That's all I was thinking, sir.'

'Quite,' Warton said, 'except he's our last bloke, and we've steadily overlooked him. And it turns out that he's a bloody genius at timing. In every case so far he's made the clock work for him – in this one, of course, quite literally. What's different now is that another clock is in play. One he couldn't know about and doesn't know about. Digestive clock. *Our* clock. Once we've got the Arab's movements confirmed, that's the one we read the time by.'

The Arab was Abo's servant. His account, that he had watched his master eat the sandwich immediately before he left, had not varied. What needed confirming was the time when he had left. The last bit of evidence on this came while they were still sitting there.

The man had said that on leaving the flat he had walked across Sloane Square to a mansion in Eaton Square where three other Arabs had been waiting for him in the servants' quarters to begin a tournament of backgammon. Each of these Arabs had now been questioned and had given, to within a few minutes, a time of arrival for Abo's man of six-forty-five.

The distance between the flat and the Eaton Square house had been paced out with him and gave a timing of thirteen minutes; which gave a sandwich time of roughly six-thirty, and a time when digestion of it had ceased at between seven and seven-thirty.

It was between seven and seven-thirty that an alibi was needed now.

It was between these times that Colbert-Greer didn't have one.

Warton carefully read out his statement.

Colbert-Greer had had an appointment at Shaft at nine o'clock, but because he'd finished his work early and needed exercise he had gone for a walk. He wasn't sure what time it was, but it was a raw evening so he'd walked fast. He thought he'd turned in to The Gold Key somewhere round about eight o'clock ('almost exactly dead on eight,' Warton said), where he had found friends and where he had become, he was sorry to say, the weeniest bit pissed. This had caused him to remain there till nine-thirty.

A few questions had been put to Colbert-Greer after his statement. He'd been asked if he had received any phone calls just before he left, or had heard his phone ringing as he went out. After a thoughtful pause he had said he hadn't. He had been asked if anyone might recall having seen him during his lengthy walk. With no pause at all he had jauntily replied that since it was dark and cold and every other pedestrian in the street walking just as briskly, he doubted it.

'Well, that's it,' Warton said. 'Same sort of thing we've always had from him. Perky. Always leaving a few vague loopholes to be investigated. Investigate them, and you find he's in the clear. In the clear on the loopholes, that is. And only vague about them. On vital timing he's always been careful.'

He briefly recapped some earlier bits of timing.

For Wu's murder, his alibi had been the Indian. But he had been the one who had carefully told the Indian the time.

Shortly after the Dutch girl's murder – within minutes of the attack on little Steve – he had coolly presented himself for his appointment with Steve. He had kept this appointment bang on the dot, though he'd apparently walked all the way.

At the time of the present murder, supposedly at eight, he had been getting himself 'the weeniest bit pissed' in a highly public place.

'It's always been important to him, timing,' Warton said, 'and I take blame for not spotting it.'

He gave the reasons for this. He had simply never been able to view Colbert-Greer as capable of murder. And he thought that from the very first interview Colbert-Greer had spotted it. His manner had certainly changed. He had become cocky, roguish, consistently over-stressing his sexual ambiguity, even his deviance with regard to drugs.

He had cheekily let them find the small quantity of marijuana. The manner in which he had allowed this to happen, in which he had allowed them to find the sketchbook – the whole life style he had exhibited for them – had shown a general feckless-ness, surely unlikely in the cool and collected murderer they were looking for. Only with hindsight was it possible to see this feck-lessness as in fact recklessness; a controlled recklessness, of the kind predicted by the psychiatrist.

The sketchbook, Warton thought, had been designed to lead them to Artie Johnston. And it looked as if Artie had cottoned on to this. He had certainly at some point become suspicious of Colbert-Greer. As had been noted – he nodded at Mason, whose observations were now in the Journal – he had steered clear of him at the gay club.

On Artie himself, he thought much of their earlier thinking could still stand. He had certainly been at Wu's cash-box, with Steve Giffard; had probably taken something from it. Just as probably he had mailed the something to Liverpool, and had gone up to dispose of it. But he doubted now if he'd mailed the lot, because he doubted if they'd found the lot. Someone had been at Wu first, and presumably also at his cash-box; had perhaps cunningly left in the box just about the sum so urgently needed for the film.

Artie's subsequent movements, suspicious at the time, had proved innocent enough. His sudden dash to the restaurant had been only to collect his copy of the shooting script, left in the confusion of the late night before, and needed for technical work on the film. All his sudden trips about London of the past few days had been found to concern only the film.

On Steve Giffard the record was less straight. The only timing for him was his monitored phone call to Artie. It was an exact timing, however, and both it and the transcribed contents seemed to clear him beyond reasonable doubt. It was virtually impossible for him to have nipped over to the Arab's, done everything that had been done there, and return inside half an hour; apart from the fact that his arm was in a sling. Of course, the arm could have been taken out of the sling – his wounds must be on the mend – but for any credible view of him as a suspect too many things were lacking.

'Mainly in the department of inches,' Warton said. 'Switch that thing on again, Summers.'

Summers switched on the video and the four men watched. They ran it several times, watching in particular the booted feet to see if anything in that quarter might be helping in the department of inches. But nothing was. The rubber boots were normal, and the masked figure walked normally in them. The huge wig made exact assessment difficult, but allowing for essential anatomy below, especially the eyes, they were able to agree on height.

'It's six-footers and over we're after,' Warton said, 'and we've only got two, and one of them we know it can't be.'

'Pull in Colbert-Greer, sir?' Summers said.

'No. The bloke was wrong, not the strategy. I want a double tail on him. I want a double tail on all three.'

'All three?' Summers said, blanching. 'That's eighteen men.'

'That's right,' Warton said, and mused. The character they were after was as elusive as a butterfly, with a habit of fluttering away under your hand; as under the hands of the man in Oxford Street a thousand years ago. To be certain of a win at the three-card trick, and wasteful as it seemed, you had to put your money on all three.

32

AT the time that the tails went on him, Frank was up in the reference library, sniggering. Brenda found him at it when she went in to tell him it was a quarter-past five. She did this not as a courtesy to him, but because she'd just had a phone call asking her to.

He seemed to be laughing over a number of copies of something, which he swept together quite briskly and put in his pocket.

'Are you going to clear up all this mess, then, before you go?' Brenda said.

'Darling, I'm going to clear up a lot of messes before I go,' Frank told her. 'Just you wait and see when my book comes out,' he added.

'I'll die of impatience,' Brenda said.

Frank looked at her thoughtfully.

'Will you, now?' he said. 'Well, that would be an interesting way to go, wouldn't it? ... How about giving the scholars a hand, then, and we'll have this little place neat as a pin in no time.'

There was something so overpoweringly sickening about him today – malicious as well as mischievous – that Brenda couldn't bear to be in the room with him.

'Okay, leave it,' she said. 'I'll do it. You go now.'

'Well, you little love!' Frank said. 'Are you sure now?'

'Positive. Good night.'

Behind Frank, as he left the library, two arms of the law took station and proceeded along Manresa Road with him, turning at the corner into the King's Road. All three of them walked to the post office, and two of them waited there while Frank went on alone to keep his appointment. It was only at Mooney's opposite.

*

All day at the *Globe* acrimony and complaint had filled the air.

'If it's laid down as a fact of nature,' Chris said, 'that Arabs are just now not in season –'

'Yes, and if one's every bloody utterance is to be treated with quite such literal –'

'And if a specific instruction is given to scrub Arabs, is it wholly reasonable to hurl charges, rebukes and seven barrels of shit if that instruction –'

'Well, what's she doing about *this* bloody Arab?'

'What we really want to do,' Mooney said, 'is give it a colossal spread. I mean, we're talking here not just about little paragraphs or news items. We're talking about a *spread* – the centre spread, with front page billing, and photos of all three of you, and frames from the film. You can surely see what's in *that*?'

'I can see what's in it for you,' Artie said. 'I don't see what's in it for us. I mean, if they've got no photos of Abo or this costume, and we do have them on our frames, and you're the only one who knows about it, a smart chick like you has to see that more than a small piece of change is involved.'

'Christ, Artie, you're small-minded. You're being offered thousands in free publicity. They'll blow up your film into a huge saleable property –'

'We don't have one, sweetie. We haven't finished it. We need the money *to* finish it.'

'And this will bring it, you barmy idiot. It will bring in dozens of people.'

'She's right,' Steve said. 'She is, you know. Only all three of us have to agree. And where's bloody Frank got to again?'

Bloody Frank was just then peering at doorbells below. One of them said *S. J. Tizack, M.Ch.S. Chiropodist. 1st Floor. Press & Enter.* The other said TOP. He pressed Top.

'Hello,' hailed a faraway voice through the battered grill from Top.

'It's Frank, Mary.'

'Okay, push . . . You in?'

'In.'

Frank went into the gloomy passage and up the stairs. Someone was howling gently in S. J. Tizack's. He carried on up the next flight, and found Mooney grimly waiting on the landing.

'Five o'clock was the time,' she said.

'Sorry, Mary. Sorry you had to ring Brenda. I lost track.'

'Well, come in and tell your producer he's a silly sod.'

Apprised of the situation, Frank gave it immediate and whole-hearted approval. 'It's a marvellous idea,' he said. 'Of course you must do it, darling.'

'Hang on,' Steve said. 'Artie has some marvellous ideas, too.'

He told Frank Artie's ideas, and Mooney answered with her own, and while doing it suddenly realized that Artie himself had stopped giving ideas. He hadn't said a word since Frank's arrival. She recalled the true purpose of this meeting; and to give herself time to think, turned away to pour drinks.

The true purpose was not the one at present under discussion. She was certain that the *Globe* would print the spread, but she didn't want them to. Not yet. She wanted no Press interest in the film story until she'd landed the main one. And the main one, she sensed, was close now.

One of these three was the murderer. And two of the three knew it; she was sure of that. She was trembling slightly as she turned with the drinks.

She let them haggle for a while on the subject of treatment and fees; waiting for the main story to come up. One of them would bring it up.

Steve did. 'Are we still under suspicion, by the way?' he said.

'Yes, all still in the running,' Mooney lightly told him. 'But only because they've got nobody else. You know how they think.'

'*I* don't, darling,' Frank said. 'They're wonders to me, those men. You mean they honestly think we're depleting the neighbourhood?'

'They know just one person is doing it.'

'Why?' Artie said. He'd livened up suddenly.

'The messages are all from the same hand.'

'*Hand-written* messages?' Steve said curiously.

'From the same person, anyway. And there's apparently nothing random in the murders. They've had accurate warning each time.'

'Have they actually told you that?' Frank said, fascinated.

'Not for publication. But another thing they know is that the victims were all quite well known to the murderer.'

'Well, they were certainly known to us,' Frank said.

'That's why you're all in the running.'

'Is it why they're searching again?'

'Who's searching?' Mooney said.

'The police. I've got a bank box in Lombard Street – a few things of my father's. They went through it again today.'

'Did they tell you?' Artie said.

'They didn't. A chap at the bank did – on the phone this afternoon.'

Artie stared at him.

'I thought you were at the library all afternoon,' he said.

'Well, I called him. Had to pop out: another matter. But there it is. Still at it, you see.' His eyes were mischievous behind the glasses. 'Could it be numbered dollars, do you think?' he asked Artie.

Artie didn't reply, but Mooney did. 'They're after a lot of things,' she said. 'And they're looking in a lot of places.'

Steve took his arm from the sling and gently eased it. 'Maybe that explains this,' he said. With the other hand he rummaged in his pocket and brought out the *Chelsea Gazette*. ' "Land-ladies warned of artful lodger",' he read, as he unfolded it.

Mooney felt her cheeks grow hot as he read out the report. But his eyes were on the paper, and the eyes of the other two were on him. Mooney kept her eyes on all three, and saw no flicker of reaction.

'So what!' Artie said, when he had finished.

'They seem to think he has another room somewhere.'

'Well, what will they think of next?' Frank said, looking at his watch. 'If that's the lot, gentlemen, and lady ... Pressing social engagements, you know.'

'We'll settle Mary first,' Steve said.

They'd already settled the outlines of the story, so the only question remaining was financial. They settled that the *Globe* had to do better than £500. 'Which is still a lousy deal,' Artie said. 'But for a fast one we'll take it.'

Mooney said she'd try for a fast one, and waited on the landing till she heard the door below slam behind them. Then she went to the kitchen and opened the gas oven. The tape recorder was running quietly inside.

She took it out and listened to a few minutes of the conversation, blinking rapidly.

She still couldn't be certain which of them it was.

All she knew was that the story of a lifetime was here. It was almost ready for hatching now.

She gave them a few more minutes to get clear of the place, and then put on an anorak and descended through the now empty building. Her bike was in a cubby hole behind the stairs. She manhandled it, swearing, through the narrow front door, and took off on her evening's mission.

In view of the newspaper report, just read out, it wasn't the healthiest mission to be engaged on. But she pedalled rapidly off. Two hours wasted on the meeting – except not wasted if she found what she wanted, or even if the police found it first. Either way it was probably her last chance of seeing the three of them together.

And in this, Mooney was right. It was her last chance.

She had a blank night on the landlady front.

33

In the night, the telex began chattering from Munich. There wasn't enough in it for the duty officer to disturb Warton, but an early call went to him in the morning, and he drove briskly to Chelsea.

Nellie Heemskerk had been located. Further details would be supplied as soon as possible. The details began coming in as soon as he entered the Incident Room, and he sat by the machine himself, watching the words appearing on the paper.

The English was rather odd, but the sense admirably clear and methodical. Nellie Heemskerk was registered at the Munich Academy of Art. Delay in locating her was because she had gone into religious retreat for the week of Advent; she was in a small convent at the nearby village of Nymphenburg.

HAVE YOU QUESTIONED HER? Warton typed.

The machine purred and chattered back. PRESENTLY NOT. CONVENT SILENT FUR ADVENTWOCHE. IF URGENT MUST TRY MUTTER.

'Mutter?' Warton said, scowling.

'Maybe they whisper there,' Summers suggested.

'I think, sir,' Mason said, and coughed.

'Eh?' Warton turned and peered up at him. 'I thought you were on night turn, lad.'

'Just off it, sir. I think *Mutter* is German for Mother. Mother Superior.'

'Ng.' Warton got busy with two fingers. He punched out: MUCH OBLIGED. PLEASE TELL MUTTER MATTER . . . He scratched his head and started again. PLEASE TELL MUTTER THE MATTER IS LIFE OR DEATH. MUST KNOW IF HEEMSKERK HAS LETTERS FROM DEAD GIRL GROOT.

The machine purred a moment and responded. UNDERSTOOD. WILL TRY MUTTER AND ADVISE YOU.

'Efficient coppers there,' Warton said, with some satisfaction, tearing off the paper roll for filing. 'Look at this, Summers. Passport number, place and date of birth . . . Religious retreat, eh?'

He noticed that Summers was not looking at him. A slight disturbance had broken out at the far end of the Incident Room where the postal clerks were sitting. He saw a postman standing there, and went swiftly over.

They were just opening it, using Kleenex sheets. It was addressed to Murder HQ.

Warton stared at the contents, and then at Summers.

All as before: cartridge paper, four lines of Letraset Gothic.

> For every time
> She shouted 'Fire!'
> They only answered
> 'Little liar!'

'Why, that's Belloc's!' Mason said.

'Now then, Mason!' said Summers, in some surprise, having misheard the vowel.

'Hilaire Belloc. The poet. I'm sure of it.'

In Warton's room, they swiftly checked. Belloc's it was:

> For every time She shouted 'Fire!'
> They only answered 'Little liar!'
> And therefore when her Aunt returned,
> Matilda, and the House, were Burned.
> *'Cautionary Tales'*
> *Hilaire Belloc.*

Warton was silent for some time.

'Get the cards,' he said, at last.

There were no gaps in the cards this time. H.B. immediately became flesh as Mrs Hester Bulstrode. Her cards produced several other cards. All concerned the inflammation risk of a boiler on the premises.

Frank's premises.

'Damn it, he can't get much nearer the wind!' said Summers.

Warton brooded a long time.

'I am not pulling him in,' he said. 'I am not! The Yard can go and take a running –'

He heard Summers coughing, and looked up to find him glancing significantly at Mason.

'Okay, lad. Get off,' Warton said.

'If there's anything I can –'

'Get off.' His head was down, menacingly low.

After Mason had gone, he said, 'Where was it posted?'

'New King's Road, sir. Not a hundred yards from his house.'

'When?'

'After four. That was the last collection.'

'And the tails went on at five, eh?'

'That's it.'

'Timing, you see,' Warton said. 'Well, Jesus Christ.'

'Yes, sir.'

'Playing with us. Wants us to pull him in. Why?'

Summers blew down his pipe.

'I am bloody not doing it,' Warton said with soft violence. 'End of the day, he'll be laughing at us . . . Where is he?'

'Got a lecture at the art school this morning, sir.'

'Check the house, then. Use the earlier complaint.'

'And inform the Yard?'

Warton quietly swore. 'Tell them, and the decision's not ours.'

'It doesn't have to be this charge, sir. There's the marijuana.'

'I know it. So does he . . . What the hell is he playing at?'

He stared hard at the few lines of type, trying to will the meaning.

'He's got something going, Summers. Pull him in, and it will happen then.'

'Can't leave the old lady at risk, sir.'

'He's figured that . . . Anything with the bloody landladies?'

'Not yet, sir. It's still early.'

Warton sat hunched and smouldering.

'We're being crowded, Summers. Being directed into this.' He could see the slug on the soil, and his own finger directing it to the bait. 'It's a fix. And just when things are going for us. Well, goddam it – if he tries to go back, take him in. Have to.'

'Yes, sir.'

'Meanwhile give Munich a nudge every hour. And watch the bloody mail. There's a landlady somewhere, Summers.'

'Somewhere,' Summers said.

All morning he watched the mail, and sent a party to the house, and every hour gave Munich a nudge; and to his relief was not prodded into action on the Colbert-Greer front. After his lecture Frank went to the British Museum; and the boiler turned out to be in perfect condition, and Munich grew increasingly irritable at the nudges.

Late in the day they came up with information, however.

HEEMSKERK HAS LETTERS FROM GROOT. SHE AGREES RETURN MUNCHEN MORGEN. NEEDLESS YOU CALL. WE CALL YOU MORGEN.

'Morgen, eh?' Warton said. 'Well, he'll stay here till Morgen.'

Frank was below in the lockup. At five o'clock he'd tried to go home. Scotland Yard had been informed. Marijuana was the charge. He didn't seem unhappy.

That was the situation at seven o'clock when Mooney found the room.

*

She couldn't all at once believe it. It was Tuesday, her late day, and she'd raced through it to start again. Right away, at the very first house, Sevastopol Street, it had happened. She'd been there twice already, without raising the landlady, a Mrs Ruddle. She didn't raise her this time, either. An old fellow with a pipe, evidently Ruddle, came to the door.

'I was wondering,' Mooney said, 'if the room was still available.'

Ruddle took his pipe out. 'Well, you're quick,' he said. 'Did you get it from the card?'

The card took a minute or two to work out. He'd apparently put one in the window of a local newsagent's that morning.

The Biffy routine took longer.

'Biffy?' he said and stared at her. 'Would that be Mr Freer, then? ... Skinny chap, glasses, pops in and out.'

'It could be,' Mooney said, with her heart lurching. 'Is he – is he in *now*?'

The man glanced briefly down the passage, apparently at a fanlight, before turning back. 'No, he's gone. Went yesterday.'

'Yesterday! Was he the – did he apply for the room after an advert in the *Gazette*, three or four weeks ago?'

'That's right. He didn't use it much, but –'

'Can I come in?' Mooney said.

'We're a bit untidy. The wife's ill, and –'

'What – 'flu?' Mooney said, sympathetically prodding him inside. 'And looking after yourself, I expect, poor man.'

'Well, I am, but –'

'Oh, this is nice. Homely,' Mooney said, looking around with approval at the fairly stinking little hovel. Rotting antlers abounded on discoloured walls.

'*Who is it?*' gurgled an old voice from above.

'For the room!'

'*Well, tell them – tell them –*' came the voice before subsiding into a terrible fit of sneezing.

'It's not convenient now,' the old chap said.

'But since I'm here,' Mooney said, 'I'd just love a peep.'

'You see, it's not actually –'

'*Fred – tell them – tell them –*'

'You keep quiet, Mother! I'll be up. Anyway, it's gone,' he told Mooney, 'so there isn't any point.'

'Gone? But you just put the card in,' Mooney said.

'I shouldn't have done. The wife had took a deposit, which I didn't know. Came in the post. And now the letter's gone off, and we have the cheque, so it wouldn't be right.'

'But I'm *here*,' Mooney said indignantly. 'And what's a deposit? He probably sent twenty others. That cheque could be stopped by now.'

'Eh?'

'Easily. There's a lot of it going on.'

'But – it's untidy, anyway, what with the wife –'

'I could have a *peep*, couldn't I, get an idea? Which one is it, first along?'

'No. Second. But I –'

'*Fred – Fred – tell them it's – it's –*'

'You keep still, Mother!'

You bloody freeze, Mother, Mooney silently advised. 'What – this one?'

'Yes, but –'

'Oh, it's just right,' Mooney said, briskly opening the door and switching on the light. And so it was. The first glimpse, the first sniff, had told her. A faint sweetish smell hovered about the place, with something rather cloying and acrid behind it. The room had been left in a hurry, a door of the rickety wardrobe ajar, one drawer of a lopsided chest still open. The bed was made up but apparently unused.

'Just like him. Always in a hurry. Popped in and out, did he?'

'Yes. Funny customer. His room, of course, so he could do what he liked with it, but – Oh, sorry. Your friend.'

'No. He *is* funny,' Mooney said firmly. 'I wouldn't even know how to describe him. How would you?'

'Well, he didn't sleep here, so I never met him.'

'But your wife's surely –'

'*Fred – Fred!*' came the old gurgle, now in considerable rage. '*I want you – I want –*'

'You see, it isn't convenient now,' Fred said.

'Well, I'll just jot my name and address,' Mooney said, 'while you see what she wants. I'll be all right here.'

'Well, I –'

'Is there a lemon in the house?'

'A what?'

'Her throat. I can hear it. Or tea with a spot of something in it. No milk. See if she wants it. I'll be here.'

'Look, I don't want to be rude –'

'*Fred – are you – are you – bloody* deaf, *Fred? I want –*'

'You'll have her up all night, you know,' Mooney said, pursing her lips and shaking her head, 'unless you see to her, for goodness' sake.' She had begun slowly writing Mrs Tizack's name and Mrs Thatcher's address.

Fred was looking somewhat flummoxed as he set off in the direction of the bronchial explosions. Mooney set off on a rapid circuit of the room.

Wardrobe empty. Chest of drawers empty. Nothing under the pillow, mattress, or bed. The acrid element in the smell seemed to come from below a small table near the curtained window. A small metal bin stood there. There was ashtray rubbish and burnt paper in it.

She looked rapidly about for something to pour it into. There was nothing in the room, so she swiftly opened her handbag, and just at the last moment paused. A few sizeable bits of paper were at the bottom of the bin, parts of a sheaf that had been torn in quarters and burnt; not evidently thoroughly enough. She picked out fragments that came whole and had them in her bag by the time the footsteps returned.

Fred was in a tougher frame of mind on returning.

'You'd better go now,' he said. 'And the milkman cashed that cheque, same time as he took the letter to the post for the wife, so no problem there. If you want to leave a name and address you can. But they go like hot cakes, these rooms, so a deposit would be better.'

Mooney said she thought she'd just leave her name and address; and inside a couple of minutes was pedalling home. The few words she'd made out on the paper indicated that Fred's lodger was a funny customer indeed.

She put the fragments together on the kitchen table and sat and pored over them. A large irregular hole had been burnt out of the middle, but the drift was clear enough:

> *Dear Sirs,*
> *I am not a racist and have never held with*
> *sending the blacks*   *believe*
> *in live and*   *have to*
> *learn how to*   *like toilets*
> *and dustbins*   *one*
> *here who dumps*   *not*
> *right. I see*   *Colston*
> *Street, bottles &*   *carnival*
> *mask, like children*   *is a*
> *Big Head (!!!) and*   *no*
> *talking, so it is for the Authoroties and not*
> *ordinory Respectible People to See him Off.*
>   *An Englishman and Proud of It.*

Three of the fragments were the same; earlier or later attempts. The thing was a draft: word order identical, the only difference in hand-writing or spelling. Fred's lodger had worked carefully to produce a semi-literate accusation against someone; against a black from the Colston Street area.

Artie lived in Colston Street.

Mooney saw the pattern suddenly, and it wasn't such a terrific surprise, but her heart was thumping so she gave herself a stiff brandy before calling Artie.

There was no reply from Artie, so she tried the restaurant. The restaurant said Artie wasn't working that night. She hung up, and tried Steve. There was no reply from Steve.

All this time Frank was in the lockup but Mooney didn't know it, or the matter might have seemed less urgent to her. As it was she gnawed her nails and tried out a few intros for the story of a lifetime; and at half-hourly intervals tried the pair again.

But she gave up at one o'clock and went to bed, her brain racing. On this night of all nights, where the hell were they?

On this night Steve and Artie had suddenly, almost unbelievably struck lucky. Isaacs, the distributor, had a colleague in town from Los Angeles. In the afternoon he'd organized a showing of what they'd done so far, and the man was crazy about it. 'Oh, the kids will love it!' he exclaimed.

He had become so expansive he'd invited them to dinner, and after dinner he wanted to see it again.

Isaacs had a small projection room at his home in St John's Wood, and around midnight they'd sat and watched it again. Artie was by now very nervous and too ready to explain some of the shortcomings, but the man had cut him off. 'Kiddo, relax. You've really *got* something – a whole new line of gags. What do you need for completion?'

In the cab going home, Artie said, 'Am I dreaming?'

'Am I?' Steve asked. 'I'll tell you one thing – that's where the heroes come from.'

The hero had guaranteed them completion. He'd put down ten thousands dollars already. After the sums they'd worked with, it was almost overkill.

*

Very early in the morning, Mooney got Artie.

He couldn't at first understand what she was talking about.

'What time is it?' he said.

'Seven o'clock.'

'Shit, I've hardly slept. *What's* so urgent?'

'I can't tell you now, but believe me it is.'

He was blinking himself awake. On his bedside pad he'd made a few notes before hitting the pillow.

'Make it at one, then,' he said. He had nothing for one, lunch-time. The pad was solid both sides of one. Ten thousand to spend!

'*One?* Look, I've got to see you right away!'

'Sugar, right away I'm going back to sleep. Is one good or not? It's all I've got.'

'Artie,' Mooney said recklessly. 'Someone is fixing you.'

'For what?'

'You know . . .'

'Oh, Jesus,' Artie said crossly. 'Mary, I'm through with all that. You know the pigs are on this phone? Do you want one o'clock or not?'

'Okay, I'll have it. At my flat.'

'But I'll be in town then.'

'*Please* Artie. At my flat!' Where the tape recorder was.

Artie stroked his great globe. 'Well, okay,' he said. 'And I got news for you, too. A better story, baby.'

'Great,' Mooney said, and hung up and called Steve.

It took longer to get Steve.

He seemed slightly stupefied when he came to the phone.

'You what?' he said.

'I've already spoken with Artie,' she repeated, 'and he knows the urgency. He'll be here by one.'

'Well, okay . . . I mean, Christ, Mary. It's a bit early now, isn't it?'

'Listen – is this line all right?'

'The line?'

'Is it bugged?'

'Bugged?' he said stupidly. 'I don't know. The whole hostel uses it. What are you talking about, Mary?'

She said, 'Steve, don't – just don't tell Frank about this. I can't – Look, be here.'

'Where?'

'At my flat!' she said. She wanted to shake him. 'At one o'clock. Have you got it?'

'I think so. At your flat. At one. Okay.'

'Be here!' she said.

There were a thousand things to do. The *Globe* had to be alerted. Art department: photos of the house. If enough people were available it might be possible to find where the 'carnival mask' had been dumped in the Colston Street area by 'the black'. There was a bio to be written; also one on his famous father. Oh boy!

Rapidly sluicing herself under the shower, Mooney thought of all this, and was glad it was still early.

34

MRS HESTER BULSTRODE awoke early, wondering if it was her bladder that had wakened her, or the strange smell in the room. Her hand groped for the transistor and switched it on.

'. . . has again called for union support in its policy of pay restraint. And the weather men promise more rain.'

Yes, and so they might. It was going cats and dogs out there, she could hear it. Maybe that had affected her bladder. She urgently rose, shrugged herself into dressing-gown and slippers and shuffled out of the room, transistor in hand.

She had her own little bathroom, but there was no lavatory in it. She'd asked the Indian fifty times, had shown him where one could go, wouldn't mind paying a bit extra for it. And much he cared! She still had to use the public one in the hall. At her age.

She remembered to shoot the bolt, and sat and listened to correspondents sounding off from all over, Washington, Moscow, Tel Aviv. God knew what they were all up to in the mad world. The only improvement in it was her transistor, which at least let her know things were no better elsewhere.

It hadn't really been so urgent, her bladder.

It must have been the funny smell in the room, then.

She could still smell it, although it was fainter.

Strange. The men had come and looked at the boiler yesterday, and hadn't found anything wrong with it. Must be something wrong with her nose.

She sniffed and pulled herself together and returned to her room.

She could definitely smell it. Stronger now. Was it petrol?

She couldn't ask the men back again. Not after they'd just been. She wondered if anyone else could smell it.

No use asking that Colbert-Greer above. The pansy.

She got back in bed and tossed and turned restlessly.

A chap was going on about Bangkok.

Anyway, the young pansy above wasn't there. She could usually hear his bed creak. She hadn't heard him last night, either. She never got to sleep herself till about two, dozed and woke; but she always knew when he was there. Him and his boyfriends. What a world.

There was a man going on about the world food situation.

She suddenly remembered, a faint crumb of pleasure, that she could make herself a bit of toast for breakfast this morning. The grill hadn't worked for weeks, but the pansy above had fixed it for her. He'd told her not to use it till today. Maybe he wasn't so bad after all ...

She dozed off, still sniffing, knowing it must be her nose, wondering if she'd feel like breakfast, anyway.

Frank had porridge for breakfast and sent his compliments to the chef. 'I've not had it since nursery days. Very tasty,' he told the solid fellow in blue, 'and just the stuff for lads. I must get his recipe.'

He was in good spirits, and only regretted that they'd given him a rather hard nylon toothbrush. 'Have to watch one's toothy-pegs,' he'd told this same fellow, who had very slightly bared his own at the remark. 'But when am I going to see your Superintendent?'

He had made it sound as if the duty of the official named was to watch them rather than him.

But for this meeting, though he remained cheerful – knowing they'd find nothing, at least of the kind they so paramountly hoped to find – Frank had to wait.

Even earlier Warton had been alerted to the additional evidence now very rapidly building up.

*

The clock was an hour earlier in Munich and the stuff had started coming through before the last shift was off. The duty inspector had called Warton, and read the message. The subject Heemskerk (born, etc., passport number, etc.) had been driven back to Munich late the previous night and was going through her papers. They would be transmitted when available.

Before he left home, Warton had phoned in himself, and had found one of his own inner team reliably there. The fellow had noted that the stuff was coming through in Dutch and had already made arrangements to have a Dutch translator on hand.

There was an air of solid business when he arrived; Summers now there and assembling the material.

'There's no stopping them, sir,' he said. 'They're sending every bloody word she ever wrote.'

Grooters had written seven letters to her friend Nellie, all of which she had kept, and all of which were being painstakingly transmitted, with frequent breaks for repetition of uncertain passages; the language unfamiliar to the man at the other end of the telex.

Warton cast an eye over the early pages as he sipped his coffee. It was coming in sheet by typed sheet from the translator in the Incident Room.

Grooters was happy to say she felt a perfect Londoner. She had a quaint flatlet in an old English mansion that had belonged to a Sir Arthur Comyns – the Comyns Hall of Residence in the address. The Albert Bridge Road was named after Prince Albert, the husband of Queen Victoria, and she could actually see the bridge, gracefully spanning the Thames and beautifully lit up like a Christmas tree. At the art school everybody was most helpful and courteous in the English manner ...

'Ng ... How's the mail?' Warton said.

The mail was productive, too. Three of the landladies approached through box numbers had replied. One had returned the cheque, another had kept it as a deposit, saying that rooms were frequently available since the house was conveniently close to the West London air terminal.

'West London? A bit far out,' Warton said. 'How's that?'

'This particular ad. went in all editions, sir. Eight papers.'

'Unlikely . . . What's this?' He was looking at the third.

It was headed *67, Sevastopol Street*.

It was signed *N. Ruddle (Mrs)*.

'That one,' Summers said, 'seems to me a possible, sir. Between Albert Bridge Road and the power station – rundown area.'

Warton carefully read it.

As he did so, he felt the thing almost move in his hands, like a water-diviner's rod.

He suddenly knew it was going to happen today.

N. Ruddle of Sevastopol Street said that a room had that day suddenly become available.

Yes, the clever bastard had seen the Press story; had got the point. So the room had suddenly become available. One jump ahead. Not a very long jump.

The phone rang while he was reading, and Summers answered and handed him the receiver. 'Commander, sir.'

'Yes, George,' Warton said, certain now that more was on the way; the bastard no doubt throwing crackers in all directions.

'Ted, does Colston Street mean anything to you?'

'Colston Street?' He could see Summers nodding at him; but knew himself all too well. 'Yes,' he said, 'Johnston lives there. The black.'

'He does, eh? Well, get a car there fast.'

'What's –'

'Anonymous letter. Don't waste time. It's on the way to you now.'

'Okay,' Warton said, and hung up, and gave Summers the instruction; and with Summers out of the room, re-read the letter. Then he got up and found Sevastopol Street on the wall map.

Yes. Had to be. Dead right. Between the power station and the Albert Bridge Road. He saw the whole thing shape suddenly.

Summers came in, and so did the letter from the Yard.

Illiterately addressed:

> *Rubbish Dept.,*
> *Police Force,*
> *London (Scotland Yard).*

Inside, a similarly illiterate scrawl.

Dear Sirs,
I am not a racist and have never held with sending the blacks back were they come. I believe in live and let live. A thing they have to learn how to use varous things like toilets and dustbins. I sorry to say we have one here who dumps his stuff all over which is not right. I see him dump yesterday in Colston Street, bottles & Things also like a carnival mask, like children they are, and this one is a Big Head (!!!) and I know for sure there is no talking, so it is for the Authoroties and not Ordinory Respectible People to See him Off.
                                        An Englishman and Proud of It.

He looked at the envelope again.

Postmarked the day before yesterday.

So had the H.B. letter been.

But that one had been sent first-class mail which had meant he would get it yesterday.

This one had been sent second-class – and to the nonsense-sounding department at the Yard – which had meant he wouldn't get it till today.

After Colbert-Greer was safely in the lockup.

He brooded over this.

'What's he got to say today – below?'

'Asking to see you, sir.'

'Is, eh? Where's Artie.'

'Tailed from his home ten minutes ago, sir . . . That car ought to be at Colston Street by now.'

'Okay. Handle it. You'll need more people. Want it gone through with a toothcomb, that street – any kind of rubbish tip, empty house, things like that. If they find anything, go yourself, immediately.'

215

'Right, sir.'

Warton had himself hooked up, on his corner speaker, so that he could listen to the operation; and he sat and smoked, hearing the cars and his Incident Room crackling away to each other in short bursts, and reading yesterday's reports, also this morning's; as well as the fresh sheets that came from the translator.

He saw that Grooters had not approved of the clay-modelling at Chelsea Art School. Pages later, she'd at last laid hands on hammer and chisel. Pages after that, she had developed a sudden interest in art history. The lecturer was amusing, the son of the famous portraitist (wrongly spelt, Colbert-*Grere*). He was acquainted with Dutch art and often spoke with her.

About ten-thirty he suddenly heard it on the speaker.

Summers looked in to say he was on the way.

They had found it: quite a haul.

Minutes later, the absolute clincher came: from next door. It was so perfect, he could scarcely believe it. He had the date of the letter checked again. But the sense was so clear, it could hardly be in doubt.

He saw the bastard still had room to wriggle, though.

He let events take their course. He left him on his own.

35

THE plain car took Summers rapidly to Putney.

He didn't spend long there. The house was one of a terrace, windows boarded up, elderly privet hedge overgrown. It totally masked the tiny front garden. A good deal of rubbish had been tipped over the hedge. A scattering of it had been disturbed to cover the deposit now disclosed.

Summers satisfied himself and left it guarded, and got through directly to Warton, who gave him fresh instructions.

At his end, Warton had the light-headed feeling of a tightrope walker, swaying with his pole, the end clearly in sight. Only a step or two to be taken now.

Mrs Bulstrode always felt a bit light-headed when she got up. The earlier rising had done nothing to mitigate this. She had felt dizzy as she'd dozed off again, and now, brushing her teeth in her little bathroom, she had to hang on to the towel rail. She put her teeth back in the glass and closed her eyes.

Oh God, it was no fun being old.

Some of the young kids on the wireless had sung a song about it, in the cynical way they had. They called themselves – what was it, The Rolling Stones yes – and although she'd felt awful at the time, she'd had to laugh. 'What a *dra-ag* it is getting *o-old*,' they'd sang. She'd actually just been sick when she'd heard it. She had been so faint she'd plonked herself down on the bed, and the little transistor had brayed from practically underneath her like a long and melodious breaking of wind.

'What a *dra-ag* it is getting *o-old*!'

But she'd had to laugh.

They did make you laugh, young people.

Some just made you sick, of course.

The dizziness was easing, and she cautiously opened her eyes.

She ought to eat something. She never felt like much, these days: tea and bread and butter. The thought of doughy bread and butter made her queasy again, so she stopped thinking of it.

Then she remembered about the grill, and a tiny miracle of appetite flared.

Well, now.

She got her teeth out of the glass and prepared to get some use out of them.

*

There were no spaces in the narrow street, but Summers had had a word with the little busybody who was writing out parking tickets. He waited double-parked till Artie came briskly out of the Soho costumiers, and then arrested him.

His orders were to arrest him only if he resisted, and he did resist. Artie was like a wildcat in the police car. Summers told him he would handcuff him if he didn't pack it in, and he was in a state of sullen silence as they turned into Colston Street.

They got him out of the car and went behind the overgrown hedge. Summers asked if he could identify anything there.

Artie said he couldn't.

'Now, then,' Summers said, 'you've already described that mask, you know you have. That's the missing one, isn't it?'

Artie said he didn't know.

He didn't know about the cape, either, or the rubber boots, or the bottle of chloroform or the cleaver.

Still on instructions, Summers took him in.

He took him directly to Warton.

Artie's face had a bluish tinge, and Warton's a yellowish one. He sat hunched in his chair and regarded Artie for a long time.

'All right, sit down,' he said.

'I'll stand.'

'Suit yourself. Cigarette?'

'Up your pipe,' Artie said.

Warton lit one himself. 'You've been had, cocker,' he said, through the smoke. 'You've been done.' He fumbled on his desk and produced the letter for Artie, and the envelope: *Rubbish Dept., Police Force* . . .

He watched Artie read it.

'Any thoughts?' Warton said.

'No.'

'Artie,' Warton said, quite mildly, 'I'm not leaning on you. You've been had, son. I know it. That cleaver, apart from anything else, was supposed to finger you. See that?'

'I don't see anything,' Artie said.

'How long do you think it would take me to find out if a cleaver was missing from anywhere special?'

'Go and find out,' Artie said.

Warton watched him for a while.

'Oh, sit down, for Christ's sake,' he said. 'You're making me nervous . . . Listen, I'm not asking you to shop him. I just want you to answer a few simple questions. Smoke if you want, you bloody fool!'

Artie accepted a cigarette and smoked it, which Warton took to be a good sign; but when he asked Artie the simple questions and Artie told him to go and fug himself, he realized it was going to take a little longer.

He said, 'Look, I'll speak plainly. I've not talked to him today, and I won't, until I've had it out with you. Try and understand what I'm saying. *You have been under constant surveillance.* Your phone has been tapped. Probably you know this. *We* know you couldn't have dumped that stuff. I am not sure that he knows it. Are you following me, Artie?'

Artie didn't bother answering.

Warton lit another cigarette.

'I'll put it another way,' he said. 'Just so you will know I am putting nothing over on you. There is an offence which you know I can get you for. I am not doing any deals with you. Probably I will get you for it. But this one is a lot more serious. Murder, Artie. In view of this letter, and what's been found, I am bound to hang on to you, unless you satisfactorily answer my questions. Answer them – a perfectly understandable thing to do for a man charged – and I could even let you go about your business. I know you've got plenty of business to attend to, Artie.'

Artie thought about it.

'*Are* you charging me?' he said.

'Not at the moment.'

'Then get fugged,' Artie said.

'Okay. We'll do it the long way,' Warton said.

By twelve-forty-five they were still doing it the long way.

Artie couldn't identify the costume or say if it had been altered. He couldn't say if he'd ever seen the cleaver. He had no knowledge of Colbert-Greer's sexual proclivities. He had never heard that the police had the numbers of Wu's dollars.

'Okay,' Warton said. 'And you won't have read anywhere that we've had messages about these murders, then.'

'That's right,' Artie said.

'So his sense of humour will surprise you.' He rummaged on his desk and produced a photo-copied example of it.

Sing Hey to you –
Good day to you!

He watched Artie read it. Artie was smoking a fresh cigarette, and his face didn't alter, but smoke came suddenly from his nostrils.

'Ring any bells?' Warton said.

Artie just shook his head.

'Try these,' Warton said.

> Stolen sweets
>> are always sweeter,
> Stolen kisses
>> much completer.

He watched Artie's face.

> To dance to flutes,
>> To dance to lutes,
> Is delicate
> And rare.

'Nothing?' Warton asked.

'No.'

Warton watched him for some time longer. 'I don't know what to do about you,' he said. 'What would you do in my position?'

Artie gave him his familiar piece of advice.

'Oh, bugger off,' Warton said wearily. 'Go on, get out.'

Artie blinked at him.

'I can leave?' he said.

'Fast. Before I change my mind. I'll get you, cocker,' Warton said, 'and you know what for. But this one isn't yours. Watch your step.'

Summers's face was a study in consternation when he returned after detailing a man to see Artie off the premises. He had his mouth half open, but closed it again on seeing the expression on Warton's face. He couldn't recall ever seeing a more unpleasant one there. Warton was nodding at a sheet of paper in his hand.

'This here, Summers,' he said, 'is the last thing that poor girl wrote. She posted it less than an hour before she died. Sunday. It was sitting in the box till Monday morning. Ticking away like a time bomb, and he never knew it. He *doesn't* know it.'

Summers slowly read the sheet handed to him.

... in a nice shade of pink, costing only four and a half pounds, that will go with my blue skirt. I have washed it (skirt) and will iron it after I have posted this off to you, which in any case I must do fast. The exciting thing I have left to the end –

Do you see me as an actress, Nellie? Don't laugh. I have mentioned before that he is involved also with a film. To my astonishment he told me on Friday that he had in mind a particular role for *me*. I could hardly believe it, but anyway we are going out tonight to eat & talk about it – thank goodness for new blouse. He is picking me up here in my room – my God, already it's 6.30, I must fly. All this *very confidential*, Nellie. He swore me to secrecy – there is jealousy among the people here. I could pick him up just as easily – you know he lives only on the ground floor here – but he will have colleagues visiting & does not wish them to know. Intrigue! Nellie, thank you for the money!

> Much love,
> Sonje.

'He lives on the ground floor of that hostel?' Summers said.
'Who does?'
'Three guesses,' Warton said.
In the three-card trick if you backed three, you got three.

Artie emerged into Lucan Place and saw a cruising taxi and flagged it. 'King's Road,' he said. 'Opposite the post office.'
He couldn't control his hands. On his shaking left wrist he saw it was a quarter-past one. Oh Jesus, he thought, don't let it be too late. The Letraset messages that he had just seen flickered in his mind, and he remembered the other one, just as neatly done, *God Bless This Crapper*, now in Liverpool, and done by the same hand. In the one blinding flash just now, he had seen the whole lot, every fugging step of the betrayal. And the cleaver. Oh, the cleaver. Oh, the cunning bastard, to do this to him. *Like children they are, and this one is a Big Head*. Oh Jesus, let it not be too late.
Artie clutched his hands together to stop them shaking, but they shook, and his whole body did. Not be too late, he prayed.

*

Steve had arrived quite early, in fact at a quarter to one, and he pressed the button marked TOP and said, 'It's Steve,' as Mooney's voice crackled through the grill.

'Oh. Early,' Mooney said, surprised. 'Okay, push.'

Steve pushed. He tramped up the stairs, passed Tizack's landing, and went up one more.

'Well, now,' he said.

'You can say that again!' Mooney said. She'd been in for half an hour, solidly typing. She had taken a few files from the office and had them scattered on the table in the general mess of papers. The phone rang at that moment and she answered it.

'Chris! Not yet, for goodness' sake,' Mooney said. 'I said I'll call *you* . . . Sure. You'll get it. Maybe in half an hour . . . Wow!' she said, hanging up. 'I tell you! Stand by for revelations, Steve. Do you want a drink?'

'Well, not unless –'

'I do,' Mooney said. She made two.

'Has a revolution broken out somewhere?' Steve said.

'It will,' Mooney said. 'Cheers.'

'Cheers. Where?' Steve said.

Mooney spreadeagled herself down, jeans-clad limbs straggling. 'I don't know where to start,' she said. 'I shouldn't till Artie gets here, anyway. Where is he?'

'He's in a lot of places,' Steve said. 'In a modest way we've got a news item of our own.'

'So he said. Where's Frank?'

'Is Frank coming?'

'I hope not. I mean – where is he?'

'I don't know. Isn't it his library day? What *is* it, Mary?'

'What it is,' Mooney said, taking a glug, 'is something you had better fasten seat-belts about . . . I really need Artie's reaction. Still, no harm in telling you, I suppose. Do you want a refill?'

'Okay,' Steve said.

Mooney got two refills.

'What I'm talking about,' she said, 'is a little house in a place called Sevastopol Street, which you won't have heard of, but which, by Christ, and by virtue of my office, you will, and so will everybody else. Are you sitting comfortably, Steve?'

'So far,' Steve said.

'Well, this same little house, in Sevastopol Street, is the head-quarters,' Mooney said, making three pronouncements of the phrase – she had got a bit light-headed suddenly with her second drink – 'of Murder Inc., British style. It sounds right, doesn't it – *Sevastopol* Street?'

'It does. What kind of murders?' Steve said.

'The Chelsea Murders. They were planned there,' Mooney said. 'I found it. *I* did. Together with the evidence. I mean, damn it, it's just a little house, and he had a room in it – and you could look for a year and never find it. Needle in a haystack. And I found it.'

'Well, wonderful,' Steve said. 'Why don't you get yourself another drink, and tell me about it. What evidence?'

'Well,' Mooney said, pouring her third, 'it's long and laby-rinthine, and rather wonderful.'

'Not too long?' Steve said, as he looked at his watch. It was a few minutes to one.

'I'll try and keep it short.'

It still came out long. By one o'clock, she still hadn't got to her piece of evidence. Steve was restive. 'Isn't Artie due?' he broke in.

'He said he might be late. Hang on, the best is yet to come.'

'Damn it, *show* me it. You're driving me mad.'

'Patience – So this old cow,' Mooney said, 'kept yelling and sneezing upstairs, and he kept trying to get rid of me . . .'

At ten-past one, she had actually got to the thing.

Steve quietly watched her.

'So what is the relevance?' he said.

'Christ – can't you see? If he'd *seen* this black dumping stuff in Colston Street, what's he doing writing about it in *Sevastopol* Street, a good three miles away? And trying it out in different kinds of handwriting. It's a *draft*. And if he's sent the police the finished copy, which presumably was the intention, well damn it – I've got the only link, and it's got to be him, hasn't it?'

'Yes. Well, yes,' Steve said. 'I suppose so. How about getting us some more drinks, then? And you can show me the thing now.'

'How many have I had?'

'Two,' Steve said.

'Liar. Give me your glass – well, it's almost full.'

'Top it up. Where *is* the stuff? Among this rubbish?'

'Leave that alone. That rubbish is a first class little bio of Frank and his Dad. Poor Frank – he must have flipped. Oh, well, truth comes first. Stop messing about with that stuff. You'll see it when Artie comes.'

'Don't be silly, Mary. You've worked me up,' Steve said. 'Let's have a glimpse, and you can hide it again, and I won't bat an eye when you tell it.'

'It isn't there, so keep your hands off,' Mooney said. 'It's in the drawer, you clot. Hang on.'

She gave him a drink and got the stuff out of the drawer. It was in a folder now, and she handled it delicately.

'I shouldn't be doing this,' Mooney said, 'and I know I've had one too many. Don't touch – it has to be photographed . . .'

She assembled it herself, carefully moving her drink out of the way. The paper was fragile, but she got it in order.

'These are his earlier inventions, see?' she said, showing the almost identical fragments.

'Yes,' Steve said.

'What the – what are you doing?' Mooney said.

Steve had crumpled up all the delicate fragments in his hand.

'I've got another invention here, Mary,' Steve said.

From his pocket he had taken a plastic bag.

'Steve – are you crazy?' Mooney said.

'Maybe a little. It won't take a minute, Mary,' Steve said.

She threw her glass in his face. He came at her with the plastic bag. It was something he had taken from the plastic bag. She found the bottle and hit him with it. It struck him hard on the forehead, spilling, but it didn't break, and it didn't stop him. He didn't even seem to feel it. He hadn't flinched, and he kept smiling. The wall buzzer sounded, and she tried to get to it – in a matter of seconds absolutely terrified, suddenly realizing everything, including the fact that she was half drunk and her limbs not working properly. She didn't get to the wall buzzer. He just jumped over the sofa and pinned her there. He got her turned round, facing the wall. She was bigger than him, much bigger, but he seemed made of coiled steel, and he had her round the throat with a pad over her face. She thought she knocked the receiver off its hook, but that was no good, wouldn't open the door that way, no good at all ...

Artie waited some seconds below, and tried again. He just kept his finger on the button and shouted 'Mary!' into the grill.

Oh Jesus, he thought, he was too late. But he couldn't accept that he was too late. There was too much energy shaking in him. He pressed Tizack's button, and heard the door click immediately, and pushed it in and ran up the stairs. He went past Tizack's landing and up the next flight, and banged on Mooney's door.

No sound there. Jesus.

The bastard had come and taken her away.

He pounded the door and put his ear to it. He could hear a sound in there somewhere, and pounded harder. 'Mary!' he called. Perhaps in some inner room, the bathroom ... The bastard had somehow got wind that they'd pulled him in and had run away. And Mary had waited here fruitlessly. 'Mary!' Artie called. Oh, Jesus.

He didn't know whether to break the door in.

He definitely heard something. There were footsteps. The door opened, and Steve stood there.

'Artie,' Steve said anxiously. 'There's something the matter with her. I don't know what it is.'

Steve was looking small and pale and fragile; also very frightened.

'She just passed out!' he said.

'Hello, then,' Artie said.

'Come in.'

'Good day to you,' Artie said.

'You what?'

'Sing hey to you,' Artie said.

225

'What are you talking about?'

Artie right away knocked him down. He couldn't control himself. He caught him a most colossal blow above the right eye, and, snarling, bent and picked him up and hit him in exactly the same place again.

'Artie!' Steve said.

Artie just pounded him. His intention was to smash him completely. He hit him several times in the same place, and then concentrated on the mouth and the nose. He wanted to obliterate the face. He held him with his left hand, and with the right had hit him perhaps thirty or forty times, very fast, like a piston, Steve's face turning this way and that under the blows, like a pale and tortured young St Sebastian, before the plain-clothes men, pounding up the stairs, swarmed over him.

Mr Tizack, his receptionist, and a shoeless patient watched, alarmed, from the landing below.

36

QUITE hideous in his triumph, Warton put up a virtuoso performance of courtliness and grace. 'Want to call a lawyer, ng? Don't have to say a word now if you don't want. Cup of tea, rest, take your time, ng?'

'Quike orrike, Chief,' Steve said nodding. 'Ake ik or gown.'

He nodded at Summers who was waiting to take it all down.

Teeth had gone; his face was an ill-defined mess; but the cockiness remained.

'Will have to ask you, in that case,' Warton said, studying the face more raptly, and bearing in mind future interpretational niceties, 'to sign every page.'

Okay, Guv, it's a fair cop, Steve wanted to tell him. But this was beyond him.

At about eight o'clock he began signing pages, though.

About this time, Mooney came to, and said she felt like death.

'Not death, dear,' Jack said. 'You don't feel anything when you're dead. You feel a lot now. You'll feel even more later.'

She raised a hand to her head, and a small flash immediately went off and she saw that a photographer was behind it. Blearily she observed that Chris was there, too, and also a large policeman. 'Where am I?' she said.

'That's a question,' Jack said, 'with important bearings. I wanted you to be at the London Clinic, courtesy of the *Globe*, but you're actually at St Stephen's, courtesy of the police. That man at the door, I don't know if you can see him, is a policeman. We got in first only because we love you. At the other side of the door I spotted people from the *Express, Sun, Mirror, Mail, Times, Telegraph* and *Guardian*. Also, I think, the *Evening News* and *Standard*.'

'Reuter and U.P., too,' Chris said. 'I saw them.'

The photographer said he'd noticed Keystone and A.P.

'Christ, I feel sick,' Mooney said.

'Darling, do you?' Jack said. 'Well, if I were you, when those people come in and start asking questions or trying to take photographs, I should just *be* sick. As often as you want,' he added. 'And I'm this moment going to see the administration about this scandalous state of affairs. Hounding patients in a public hospital. Try just two more to be certain,' he advised the photographer, as he set off to do this.

Mrs Bulstrode came to about the same time. She felt perky after her doze, and it struck her that she wouldn't mind beans on toast. The earlier toast had been fine. She couldn't remember for a moment where she kept her canned stuff – memory definitely going – but found it in the end. The thing in the bowl was in the same cupboard. The young pansy – she shouldn't call him that, really, since he'd been so useful – had filled a bowl with paraffin to try and ease the locked mechanism. It was the automatic bit of the grill that had stuck. The paraffin seemed to be the source of the smell so she poured it down the sink. She'd never used automatic, anyway.

At Sanderstead much later – actually at about three in the

morning – Rose, in her dressing-gown, brought Warton up a cup.

'What's that?' he said.

'Your cocoa, dear.'

'Come on, I'll have another Scotch.'

'Oh, Teddy. You've had enough.'

'What's up, Rosie?' Warton said, somewhat slurred. 'Not every day, you know! Last of that bloody rubbish, I tell you. They can stand on their heads. I tell you!'

'All right,' Rose said, not anxious to be told again, and brought him another.

'Clever little devil,' Warton said. 'Really was. Foxed me. Well, he could have foxed anyone.'

'Of course he could,' Rose said. 'Half-past three, dear. Are you thinking of going up there in the morning?'

*

Warton took the statement to the C.C. and stood by for explanation.

But there wasn't much to explain.

Most had already been explained, and a good part deduced.

Steve had got himself a photo-copy of the List of Residents and had seen what Detective Mason had seen. He had sent off his first quotation as a joke, but when it drew no response he had decided to take it a stage further.

He said his idea was to goad the police into publicizing the joke murder messages. He could foresee the huge newspaper treatment that would follow. His own joke murder film was at that time stalled for lack of funds. With the right publicity climate, the small offbeat production might easily mushroom into a timely and audacious entertainment that could bring kudos and fortune.

That had been the idea, anyway. But a number of developments had turned it into different directions.

The first was his palming, some weeks before, of what he thought was a bottle of laughing gas. This had been at the chemical laboratories where they had been discussing a laughing-

228

gas scene. In his flat he had experimentally tried a small amount and had chloroformed himself.

He decided to use the chloroform for his joke attack on Mrs Honey, and then realized he would need a disguise as well. As it happened, he already had this, too. After the night-shooting he found that he had crammed into his bag, along with things of his own, the discarded mask, and had so far forgotten to mention it.

He realized that he'd better not keep these things in his flat and that he needed an extra room.

When he got the room – perhaps even before he got it – the really major development occurred.

He said that in reply to the box number in the *Gazette* he had signed himself 'Freer', and as soon as he'd done it he felt freer. He realized he'd probably had in mind some echo of 'Greer' – Colbert-Greer: so he'd got himself a pair of plain glasses like Colbert-Greer's. And then everything had changed. In Freer he had another person, as separate from himself as the film. The film could play out any fantasy it wanted. So could Freer.

'Jekyll and Hyde, eh?' the C.C. said.

'Something like that,' Warton said. 'Codswallop of all sorts. You'll see it there. Stuff about the earthquake – how nobody cared about the thousands of dead. How they could be made to care about a couple of mystery deaths. Society sick. All a game. Ought to be shown up. By him and his mate Freer.'

Steve hadn't only seen how he and Freer could show up society. He had also seen how they could pick up some money as well as making a monkey out of the police, none of which could be bad for the film. Bad things wouldn't be his doing, anyway. Freer was the one who did bad things.

The first bad thing Freer decided to do was kill Wu.

Steve made arrangements. He had bought the supplies: cotton wool, plastic bags, rubber bands.

'In the next bit, he shows his talent,' Warton said. 'Timing.'

In the next bit, Steve had smartly knocked up the caretaker at the student hostel, told him he was back and was there a registered letter for him? There was and the man gave him it.

229

But Steve hadn't just arrived: he was just leaving. He'd got a taxi in the King's Road the moment he left the shop, and he took one immediately back. Into the bargain, he'd already visited Sevastopol Street, just behind the hostel, for his supplies.

In the King's Road, he watched the shop until Chen left and then went and rang the doorbell himself. Wu, mystified, had let him in, and the moment he was seated at his desk, Steve had taken the soaked pad out of the plastic bag and chloroformed him. As soon as Wu succumbed, trapped in his chair, he had fixed the bag over his head and left him to suffocate while he got the block and tackle.

Wu's pockets had produced the keys, and a brisk survey below the cashbox. Of the $2,500 in it, he had taken $2,000, leaving the 500 as well as the drugs against a probable police search: his idea to show that the murder was not for money – a thief wouldn't have left any – and to discredit Chen's possible hints on this score.

He'd then left by the back door, dumped the pad, posted off the dollars to Sevastopol Street, and had been propping up the bar at The Potters for twenty minutes when Artie at length arrived: all timing properly certified by caretakers and barmen.

'Class, you see;' Warton said. 'And it nearly worked. Well, it did work. But Artie loused it up.'

Artie had certainly done this. His lifting of the remaining $500 had provided a colossal and lasting complication.

The dollars had gone to Liverpool (Artie's idea), and after them had gone Artie, attracting police attention, and also something worse; something much worse, something absolutely hellish.

Years before at the art school (actually in their first year) Steve Giffard had been amused by the pious possibilities of Letraset Gothic, a quantity of which he had stolen together with the cartridge paper which was used to mount it. This had somehow hung around in his general mess of papers, and when the idea of sending the police a joke message had occurred, he had hunted it out: it had seemed right for 'The Blessed Damozel'.

Unfortunately for him, in that first year at the art school he had shared a flat with Artie. And for the lavatory of the flat he

230

had made a sign, *God Bless This Crapper*, out of the same type mounted on the same paper.

He hadn't forgotten the sign. He had thought he'd ditched it when they'd left the flat. But he hadn't. In some way it had been packed up with Artie's things and had found its way to Liverpool. And when Artie had gone up after the dollars he had found it again; and had nostalgically mentioned it to Steve when he came back.

This threw Steve into a panic.

The only links between him and the murder were the messages. He had sent the police three now (Germaine, Honey, Wu). Artie was the only one who could make the connection, and Artie was rash and capable of getting into all kinds of trouble. He thought something had better be done about Artie.

Steve was a planner and he didn't like playing things by ear. But he had to now. On a chance visit to the restaurant (a mess-up to do with editing gear) he had seen a cleaver and stolen it.

At this time he was already planning (his *alter-ego* Freer was, he said in the statement) the murder of the Arab, who had plenty of money and was messing them about. He decided to postpone this for the time being and instead to do something with the cleaver, which might at one and the same time exonerate him and implicate Artie. In pondering how to do it he recalled the registered-mail book he had signed on claiming his registered letter from the caretaker. Above his own name in the book had appeared that of a Dutch student with an apt set of initials, W. S. Groot.

'That was the money she was thanking her friend Nellie for, sir,' Warton advised. He watched the C.C. read slowly through the next half page and then turn rather restlessly back.

'His room *wasn't* searched after that murder?' the C.C. said.

'Not then, sir, no. You have to see the situation at the time.' Warton amplified it for him.

With the keys copied, Steve had slipped out to his other room in Sevastopol Street. His 'protection' was at the front so he had felt safe enough in slipping out of the back. He had picked up his kit (cleaver, cape, mask, etc.) and had returned and used them. He had deposited the major part of this kit in his bedroom wardrobe before returning to inflict the rather severe wound on himself in the doorway; and had then waited for the first caller and the police. The rest of the house had then been searched, but in the circumstances his own room had not been searched.

'I see,' the C.C. said.

Next day, choosing his moment, Steve had returned the kit to Sevastopol Street. But in the ensuing days, with his arm being treated, he had rethought the position. He was aware that he wasn't under suspicion himself now. As he had planned, Artie was under suspicion. This seemed now not such a great idea. Artie might be pulled in and confronted with the evidence of the messages, which was the last thing he wanted. This came of acting under pressure. He now thought without pressure.

The best idea was for Artie to be neutralized. Best of all was for him to be eliminated. But he didn't see his way to arranging this at the moment. So an interim idea was needed.

He had been aware from the start that the police knew that it had to be one of the three. It obviously wasn't him now, and it had better not be Artie. On the whole, it had better be Frank.

He thought he'd give Frank the Arab's murder.

He had been planning it for a long time and he liked every detail of it. But a detail came up just then that he hadn't thought of. With both of the other two being double-tailed (as he'd heard separately from them) how could either be in a position to send off one of the familiar messages to Murder HQ? Similarly, with only one arm, how could he prepare one?

The answer to both these points came from Father Christmas. In a heap of sales rubbish at the hostel he found him decorating a Special Offer from the L.E.B., lavish with order forms for toasters and hair-dryers, and complete with Freepost return envelope.

He over-stuck the envelope with the printed address of his local branch (Sloane Street) also included in the heap of bumf, and with his left hand and a ballpoint quaveringly added the superscription URGENT.

On a vacant bit of newspaper, he executed his chosen quotation HOPPITY-HOP in the same style, wrote out another envelope, to Murder HQ, and inserted the lot into the post-paid cover.

He realized that since police suspicion now rested on Artie, a likely result of his *coup* would be even more hawk-like vigilance; and he planned to make full use of it. The surveillance of Artie, properly managed, could serve to establish both his and Artie's alibis; leaving Frank, as planned, in vacant possession of Abo's murder.

On the day, Sunday, he phoned Abo and told him to put off all appointments after six-thirty because he had a piece of video pornography so special it would knock him cold. He also told him not to tell anyone, and to get rid of the servant. He knew Abo would do this.

And Abo did. Steve had turned up, with his supplies, in good time, watched the servant off the premises; and had then announced himself on the buzzer.

His first act on entering the penthouse was to ask to make a phone call, which he then did – to Colbert-Greer. The aim of this vital call was to ensure that Frank was alone and to take him out of circulation. He simply said he was calling to remind Frank they had a date at nine and that he should now leave his book (which he knew him to be working on) and settle to the lighting plan.

Colbert-Greer thanked him for the call, promised to start work on the plan which would only take a couple of hours, and assured him he had nobody with him. Steve hung up, easy in the knowledge that he had just handed out Abo's murder and ready now to get on with it.

He and Abo had gone to the video room, where he had put an empty spool on the player, seated Abo comfortably, and immediately chloroformed him from behind. He had managed this with the nylon noose he had brought with him. He said that Abo had fought like a cat, holding his breath for an unconscionably long time, but the noose over the pad had in the end done the trick; he had only had to keep one hand tight on the knot, though both hands were now in fair working order.

Inside fifteen minutes he had done all the things already known (costuming, clock, video-taping, trussing, etc.), and also a couple of things not known. He had relieved Abo of £700 and $1300 ('We've got it, sir – also Wu's two thousand'), and had had him nicely balanced on the fire escape, the air conditioning removing the smell from the video room, before calling Artie and establishing his own alibi at seven.

'He phoned Artie *from* the Arab's?' the C.C. said.

'That's it, sir.'

'But – Artie left immediately.'

'So did he. Got a cab in Sloane Square. *And* he went to Sevastopol Street first, and made it back home with minutes in hand. Cool customer.'

'I see.'

'Yes,' Warton said.

Just as well everybody did.

What followed was less coherent because Steve had been less coherent, but Warton explained it.

Steve's reckoning was that the police would have to accept Frank as the only one of the three without an alibi; and that if they did, all well and good. Before the messages came up at any subsequent stage, Artie would be out of the way. An accident would happen to Artie.

If for some reason the police let Frank go – after he had seen the messages – Artie's accident would have to happen faster. It would have to happen via the agency of Frank.

In any event there'd be no Artie.

There might or might not be a culpable Frank Colbert-Greer.

In no event at all would there be a culpable Steve Giffard. All the events could start to happen just as soon as Colbert-Greer was arrested.

However, the police hadn't arrested Colbert-Greer.

This threw Steve into a kind of stupor.

The following day, Monday, still slightly stupefied, he had gone to Sevastopol Street. On the way he'd bought the *Chelsea Gazette*, Friday's copy. The artful lodger.

Given his state of mind, and the emergency, Warton thought his ploy still quite acute: the message to the police that had more or less forced them to take in Colbert-Greer, and the accompanying one, due to arrive the following day, that had shown why Colbert-Greer might have wanted to be taken into custody.

The reasoning here was complex, and obviously not a hundred per cent, but still not bad. The man who had sent the illiterate letter was either a man who had seen a black man dump stuff, or one who had dumped it himself.

Since the black man in question was being double-tailed at the time and couldn't conceivably have dumped it, the sender of the letter had to be the second of the two characters. And since it was always possible, in view of the known suspicion between them, that Colbert-Greer had *not* known if Artie was being double-tailed, it looked as if he might frantically be trying to wriggle out of suspicion himself: establishing his innocence as writer of the letter by being in custody. There were holes in it, but material enough, at least, for the police to hang on to him.

That had been the idea, anyway, but it had rapidly been overtaken by other ideas.

Ideas had been going so fast then, nobody could keep up with them.

For a start, Mary Mooney had found the room, Tuesday evening.

(Steve had skipped from it on Monday afternoon.)

She had found the burnt draft incriminating Artie, and had managed to reach both Artie and Steve on Wednesday morning.

Steve had been the one who had got the point.

About the time that he had got it, the telex material from Munich had started coming in, unknown to him.

The evidence known to him he had then begun trying to destroy.

'Yes. Yes,' the C.C. said. 'But if he knew Artie was on the way –'

'His idea there, so far as he had one, was that when Artie arrived he'd try and pin the murder on him. He thought he *had* murdered her – she was shoved under the bed, with the bag not quite on her. In any case, he had to move so fast –'

'Yes. I see that. What I'm not clear on, Ted, is this question of six-footers.'

'Ah. That one. Ng,' Warton said. 'You'll see it there, sir. Not quite clear. Talking a bit funny. We thought he wanted something for his mouth, which was in a state. Pointing at it. His meaning was that he had been looking out of it. The mouth. Of the costume, sir. The neck of it was thick because his head was in it. What his eyes were looking out of was the mouth. It was open and smiling rather, like this,' Warton said, smiling most evilly with his own. 'The eyes in the costume were about six inches above his own. Gave him an extra six inches of height, you see.'

37

PEOPLE were shocked, of course.

Frank was horribly shocked.

Artie was practically *in* shock, for week after week, at Steve's betrayal, and all the things that he had done.

Steve was even a bit shocked himself, looking back.

Some called him a dastard, and others a bastard, but all agreed he wasn't mad; which was how he got life.

Artie just got six months.

Mooney got her job on the *Globe*.

Mason got made detective sergeant.

There were many around, of course, who said it was all very well solving the second series of murders, but how about the first?

Warton, by then into a dream job (up on the 9.30, back on the 5.30), had a proper answer for all these.

He could point to the distinguished list of unsolved crimes that constituted such a feature of police forces everywhere. He could and did say that almost everybody had prophesied a bad end for Germaine Roberts, and she had come to one. Miss Manningham-Worsley was a different case, it was true, but after eighty-two years could her end be said to be precipitate? As for Alvin C. Schuster (pretty obviously a wrong bloke), his bizarre extinction, so far from home, file still open, ensured remembrance long beyond the normal span.

In any case, it had all happened in Chelsea; and as far as he was concerned anything could happen there. He was through with the murder game, anyway. Too often, in that kind of game, he'd been led by the nose; and he thought he wasn't the only one.

MORE ABOUT PENGUINS
AND PELICANS

Penguinews, which appears every month, contains details of all the new books issued by Penguins as they are published. From time to time it is supplemented by our stocklist which includes around 5,000 titles.

A specimen copy of *Penguinews* will be sent to you free on request. Please write to Dept EP, Penguin Books Ltd, Harmondsworth, Middlesex, for your copy.

In the U.S.A.: For a complete list of books available from Penguins in the United States write to Dept CS, Penguin Books, 625 Madison Avenue, New York, New York 10022.

In Canada: For a complete list of books available from Penguins in Canada write to Penguin Books Canada Ltd, 2801 John Street, Markham, Ontario L3R 1B4.